diabetes
recipes from around the world

diabetes
recipes from around the world

jane frank

grub street | london

Published in 2009 by
Grub Street
4 Rainham Close
London
SW11 6SS
Email: food@grubstreet.co.uk
Web: www.grubstreet.co.uk

Text copyright © Jane Franks 2009
Copyright this edition © Grub Street 2009
Design by lizzie b design

A CIP record for this title is available from the British Library

ISBN 978-1-906502-06-5

Printed and bound in India

contents

acknowledgements

This book would not have got off the ground without the encouragement and enthusiasm of my publisher and editor, Anne Dolamore of Grub Street, who commissioned it, and I am very grateful to her for having faith in me and for giving me this opportunity.

A huge thanks to the people who tested the recipes for me. They included fellow nutritional therapists, diabetics, patients, friends and family. Without their help, advice and occasional criticism I would not have the confidence to launch these recipes on a general readership, but I know that they are sound and that none of them is hard to make. My especial thanks go to my husband John for patiently enduring my experiments in the kitchen; to Marion Billingham, who cheerfully ploughed through a huge pile of recipes, fed them to her husband Jim and sent me feedback on a daily basis; to Alison Cregeen who tested the soups chapter while juggling small children and a house move; to Josie Cowgill and Linda Marais who not only cooked several dishes but who made constructive suggestions and gave invaluable nutritional advice; to Lynn Alford-Burow who is always there for me; to Kay Clarke and her son Andrew who painstakingly photographed every ingredient of the recipes Kay tried; to Anita Townsend for her helpful comments and willingness to try unfamiliar ingredients; to Laura Fairweather, Sylvie Jackson and David and Eileen Row. Thank you all.

Finally, my special thanks go to all the people I know – patients, friends and acquaintances – who are living with diabetes, and especially to Henrietta Usherwood who has lived with this disease for nearly thirty years. She is a constant reminder to me that every diabetic has his or her own individual glycaemic response, and that what may have no effect on one person's blood sugar, may send that of another sky high. So I offer these recipes to her and to every other diabetic who picks up this book with the proviso that I've used the best information available to me, a non-diabetic, and hope that, not only will you and your family enjoy them, but that they will help your glycaemic control.

introduction

A diagnosis of diabetes can seem at first like a shattering blow. If you have been told you have diabetes, your first reaction might well be 'why me?' And yet you're far from being alone. Worldwide today there are approximately 200 million people with diabetes, more than two million of whom are in the UK. At least a million more in the UK alone – 'the missing million' – are thought to have diabetes but are not aware of it yet.

When you are first diagnosed with diabetes and you learn that you are going to have to live with it for the rest of your life, you may react with anger, shock or fear. This reaction is understandable. Diabetes is indeed a serious disease, but it is possible to lead a relatively normal life with diabetes, as many people throughout the world do. There are numerous international diabetes organisations such as the International Diabetes Federation, and most countries have diabetes support groups and charities such as Diabetes UK, the American Diabetes Association and Diabetes India. Help and information is available from all these bodies, and from the numerous diabetes forums and chat rooms on the internet. But the key to successfully coping with diabetes is still self-management, and the most important aspect of self-management is making healthy food choices. In this book I've collected together recipes from several different cuisines around the world, picking out dishes that will help you keep your blood glucose on an even keel as well as being nutritionally balanced, tasty and easy to cook. Some of these recipes are traditional dishes reworked to be more diabetes-friendly, whilst others are new recipes using culinary traditions from many different countries.

What Is Diabetes?

If you have diabetes, this means that there is too much glucose in your blood. This glucose comes from the carbohydrate foods in our diet, and is our principal source of energy. In a normal person, the level of blood glucose is strictly regulated by two hormones called insulin and glucagon, secreted by the pancreas. The job of insulin is to move glucose out of the blood and into the cells after a meal, while the role of glucagon is to raise blood glucose between meals if it is sinking too low. In a person with diabetes, this mechanism fails to work, and the blood glucose level stays too high. This could be either because the pancreas is making too little or no insulin, or because the cells have become resistant to insulin and fail to respond to its message. The action of glucagon is seldom impaired in the same way.

Signs and Symptoms of Diabetes

The first effect of high blood glucose levels is that glucose passes into the urine because it can't get into the cells where it is needed. This glucose makes the urine of a person with undiagnosed diabetes sweet, hence the name 'diabetes mellitus'– 'mellitus' deriving from the Greek word for honey. Because the urine is syrupy with glucose, the kidneys respond by excreting more fluid to try and dilute it. This results in the

The Three Classic Symptoms of Diabetes

- **Polyuria – frequent urination**
- **Polydipsia – excessive thirst**
- **Polyphagia – excessive hunger**

need to pass urine more frequently which, in turn, causes extreme thirst. The excessive fluid loss often causes the patient to lose weight, which may make them feel very hungry. These are the three classic symptoms of diabetes. Other symptoms include extreme fatigue, blurred vision, nausea and tingling or numbness in the hands and feet. Frequent or recurring infections and slow wound healing are also signs of undiagnosed diabetes. The symptoms are quickly relieved once the diabetes is treated, so it is important to get a diagnosis as early as possible. Early treatment will also reduce the chances of developing serious health problems.

Types of Diabetes

There are broadly two types of diabetes: Type 1 and Type 2. About 5% of people with diabetes have Type 1, while the remainder have Type 2. The two types are very different diseases with different causes and different mechanisms at work, but management of the two conditions is fairly similar.

Type 1 or Insulin-Dependent Diabetes Mellitus (IDDM)

In this type, which used to be called juvenile diabetes to distinguish it from the later-onset Type 2, the symptoms listed above usually appear quickly, over a period of weeks or even days, and must receive immediate medical attention. The person's blood glucose rises alarmingly because insulin production is inadequate or fails altogether.

Type 2 or Non-Insulin Dependent Diabetes Mellitus (NIDDM)

In Type 2, the same symptoms as those associated with Type 1 may occur, although not necessarily. However, they progress gradually, sometimes so gradually that you can have Type 2 without even being aware of it, and could remain undiagnosed for several years. One of the reasons Type 2 diabetes may not be recognised is that many of its symptoms, such as increased urination, lack of energy, weight loss,

skin infections and wounds that are slow to heal, are things that may occur anyway as a part of ageing. Type 2 used to be called senile diabetes, but it is appearing in younger and younger people, especially in certain ethnic groups.

Other types of diabetes include Maturity-Onset Diabetes of the Young (MODY), which is a hereditary form of Type 2 diabetes that occurs in young adults; Gestational Diabetes, which occurs in pregnancy and usually disappears after the baby is born; and Secondary Diabetes, which develops as the result of another condition, such as pancreatitis, cystic fibrosis or haemochromatosis. This last is an inherited disease that causes excessive amounts of iron to accumulate in the body, and is often referred to as 'bronze diabetes' because it is sometimes accompanied by a bronze colour of the skin.

Diagnosis and Tests

The most usual test for diabetes is a fasting plasma glucose test (FPG) which is done in the morning after the patient has abstained from food for at least 8 hours. After this long without food the blood glucose should be below 7 millimoles per litre (mmol/l) in the UK, or below 125 milligrams per decilitre (mg/dl) in the US. A reading above this level is considered to be a sign of diabetes, if confirmed by a subsequent test.

The Oral Glucose Tolerance Test (OGTT) may also be used. It is more sensitive than the FPG test, but less easy to administer. The patient has to drink a glucose drink after an 8 hour fast, and the blood glucose is measured immediately beforehand, then again two hours later. The second reading should be below 11 mmol/l or 200mg/dl. Another test sometimes used is the random plasma glucose test, which can be done at any time without any preparation. Diabetes may be diagnosed on the basis of a single abnormal blood glucose test if the patient has the classic symptoms.

Causes of Type 1 Diabetes

To search for just one single cause of Type 1 diabetes would be misguided, as different mechanisms may be significant in different parts of the world. What we do know is that in about 90% of people with Type 1 diabetes, the pancreas stops making insulin because the beta cells which secrete insulin are destroyed by the body's own immune system. Why this happens remains a mystery, although there appears to be a genetic predisposition which is activated by an environmental trigger.

About 10% of people with Type 1 have a genetic predisposition without an autoimmune reaction. Instead, they are more likely to have inherited certain types of white blood cells (called HLA types) which make them more at risk. But heredity is not the only factor. Studies of identical twins have shown that when one twin gets diabetes, the other twin only develops the disease in about half the cases, so there must be an environmental trigger as well.

During the last few decades, the worldwide incidence of Type 1 diabetes has been increasing significantly, by about 3% per year. This increase suggests that an environmental factor,

such as a virus, is involved. It's possible that the immune system, having fought off a virus, then turns on the beta cells because it confuses them with the virus. Type 1 has been associated with the coxsackie B virus among others.

Another environmental trigger could be food, and the most strongly implicated food so far is cow's milk, specifically because it contains insulin. Researchers in Finland have discovered that babies fed on cow's milk formula are five times more likely to develop Type 1 diabetes. The theory is that the baby's immune system makes antibodies against the cow's insulin, which then go on to destroy the beta cells in the baby's pancreas.

A recent review of global eating habits concluded that the worldwide increase in Type 1 diabetes could be associated with increased meat consumption, although no one understands what the mechanism might be.

The third possible food culprit is gluten – the protein found in wheat, barley and rye and usually as a contaminant in commercially grown oats. It is known that up to 10% of people with Type 1 also have celiac disease (intolerance of gluten), and it may be that eating gluten is also partly responsible for the onset of the disease. Both are autoimmune diseases and there appears to be a familial link. One in 20 people with a relative with Type 1 diabetes may be celiac.

It has also been suggested that vitamin D deficiency may be a major factor in the development of Type 1 diabetes in children. Diabetes is less common in those areas of the world where genetically susceptible children get adequate amounts of vitamin D, either in the diet or through exposure to sunlight.

Causes of Type 2 Diabetes

There is a range of risk factors for Type 2. Firstly, it occurs mostly in people over the age of 45, although it is now appearing in younger and younger people. Next, there is a

---

Causes of Type 1 diabetes

Known causes:
- **Genetic predisposition**
- **Autoimmune destruction of the beta cells**

Possible environmental triggers:
- **Viral infection**
- **Autoimmune reaction to:**
  - **bovine insulin**
  - **meat**
  - **gluten**
- **Vitamin D deficiency**

Risks for Type 2 diabetes include:

- **Age over 45**
- **African or Asian heritage**
- **Body Mass Index over 30 (over 25 for Asians)**
- **Blood pressure over 140/85mm Hg**
- **Parent or sibling with Type 2 diabetes**
- **Nutritional deficiencies e.g. magnesium/ chromium**
- **Poor dietary choices (diet high in refined and processed foods)**
- **History of gestational diabetes or having given birth to a baby over 9lbs in weight**

strong hereditary component – it is three to five times more common among African, Caribbean or Asian communities living in the UK, and tends to develop at a younger age in these groups. It seems that a large proportion of people in these ethnic groups have a genetic predisposition to develop diabetes if they diverge even very slightly from their traditional diet.

Obesity is definitely a risk factor. It is arguable whether obesity is the primary cause of diabetes, but there is no doubt that it nearly always accompanies diabetes. A diet high in processed foods, fat and sugar leads to obesity and therefore also to diabetes. High blood pressure is another risk factor. Lastly, if a woman has already had gestational diabetes or if she has given birth to a particularly large baby, diabetes is more likely to develop later on.

Insulin Resistance, Prediabetes and Metabolic Syndrome

Insulin resistance is the basic metabolic failure underlying Type 2 diabetes. When a person is insulin resistant, the pancreas is still making insulin but the cells do not respond to the normal amount of insulin, so the pancreas has to produce more insulin than normal to move glucose out of the blood and into the cells. Thus a person with insulin resistance may have high blood glucose and high insulin (hyperinsulinaemia) at the same time. Insulin resistance and hyperinsulinaemia are early warning indicators of the risk of prediabetes and Type 2 diabetes, or may indicate other medical disorders such as Polycystic Ovarian Syndrome. Insulin resistance may develop as a result of genetic predisposition; a diet high in refined and processed foods and lacking in nutrients; a sedentary lifestyle; consequent obesity; and finally stress. Stress uses up valuable nutrients such as magnesium. Acute stress, in which adrenaline is released, causes insulin levels to fluctuate wildly, whilst chronic high levels of the stress hormone, cortisol, lead to chronic high blood glucose.

As the body gradually loses sensitivity to insulin, prediabetes is the next step after the establishment of insulin resistance in the downward slope towards diabetes. Prediabetes used to be called impaired fasting glucose (IFG) or impaired glucose tolerance (IGT), but the use of the term prediabetes has been adopted to help people appreciate the serious nature of this metabolic condition and the urgency involved in making healthy lifestyle changes.

Metabolic Syndrome/Syndrome X/Insulin Resistance Syndrome (IRS) are all terms for the same collection of symptoms which, taken together, increase the risk not just for diabetes but also for cardiovascular disease and liver disease.

It is clear from a number of large-scale studies that the clock starts ticking for cardiovascular disease many years before a person is diagnosed with diabetes. Several large studies, including the Diabetes Prevention Program (DPP) in the USA, have showed how crucial healthy nutrition and exercise are in preventing diabetes and cardiovascular diseases in people with Metabolic Syndrome.

In fact, the DPP worked too well. The group on 'lifestyle

Metabolic Syndrome includes at least three of these symptoms:

- **A waist measurement of more than 40"/102cm in men or 35"/89cm in women.**
- **A waist to hip ratio of more than 0.95 for men or more than 0.8 for women. Asians are at risk at lower ratios.**
- **High levels of triglycerides and LDL – the 'bad' cholesterol**
- **Low levels of HDL – the 'good' cholesterol (less than 50 mmol/L in women and less than 40 mmol/L in men)**
- **Blood pressure greater than 130/85mm Hg**
- **High levels of blood glucose**
- **Insulin resistance**

intervention', i.e. healthy diet and exercise, turned out to have a 58% lower risk of developing diabetes than the control group who had made no lifestyle changes. This was felt to put the control group at an unfair disadvantage, and so the trial was abandoned.

Hypoglycaemia

Hypoglycaemia (a 'hypo') means low blood glucose, and is one of the effects of diabetes. It may seem illogical that low blood glucose is the most dangerous effect of diabetes, which by its very nature is a disease of high blood glucose. However, a hypo occurs if a person with diabetes injects too much insulin, or takes too high a dose of diabetes drugs. It may also happen if they skip a meal or delay eating, drink too much alcohol or exercise without eating beforehand. During a hypo the brain is starved of glucose, so the person may appear confused and behave abnormally. The only way to prevent the person going into a coma is to ensure that they eat some glucose immediately. Many insulin-dependent diabetics can feel the onset of a hypo before it happens and can thus avoid it by eating a glucose sweet or similar large dose of glucose.

Complications of Diabetes

Diabetes is such an important issue because of the long-term effects of the disease, which are serious, although they may take many years to appear. They include heart disease, high blood pressure, stroke and peripheral vascular disease (that is, diseases of the blood vessels outside the heart and brain). There are several complications of diabetes that develop over time. These include damage to the retina of the eye (retinopathy), which can lead to impaired vision and even blindness. Other complications are damage to the blood vessels, the nervous system and the kidneys. Studies show that keeping blood glucose levels as close to the normal, nondiabetic range as possible may help prevent or delay harmful effects to the eyes, kidneys, and nerves. The mechanism by which diabetes leads to these complications is complex, and not yet fully understood, but it appears to be the combined effects of high glucose levels, high blood pressure, high blood fats and damaged blood vessels.

If blood glucose levels are high over a long period, glucose molecules attach themselves to proteins, making them 'sticky'

Diabetes complications include:

- **Heart disease**
- **High blood pressure**
- **Retinopathy – damage to the eyes**
- **Neuropathy – damage to the nerves**
- **Nephropathy – damage to the kidneys**
- **Angiopathy – damage to the blood vessels**

so they can't function properly. This is called the glycosylation of proteins and, at the cellular level, is the ultimate cause of diabetic complications. For diabetics, the most significant glycosylation is that of haemoglobin, the molecule in our red blood cells which carries oxygen around the body. This glycosylation is measured by the HbA1c test. As all diabetics know, the HbA1c is a vital long-term blood glucose reading, and is used to predict the likelihood of complications from diabetes. It is important to achieve a score of less than 7% on the HbA1c test to reduce the risk of developing serious long-term health problems.

The Global Perspective

Why is diabetes on the increase all over the world, and why is it increasing in some countries more than others? Firstly, the global population is rising. A larger population clearly means that there will be more people with diabetes. Secondly, the population is getting older, so the number of people affected by Type 2 diabetes (normally associated with late adulthood) will rise. Perhaps the most significant changes, though, are the movement of people to towns and cities, an increasingly sedentary lifestyle and the globalisation of food supply, which combine to promote an 'obesogenic' environment in which it is harder and harder to keep slim and active. Until recently, overnutrition (in which fat and sugar account for over half the caloric intake) has generally been perceived as a problem of developed countries. However, overnutrition and its consequences are increasing even in countries where hunger is common. Recent reviews have found that obesity and the risk for chronic diseases such as diabetes are increasing in developing countries. They are now global problems, not just the problems of the rich countries. In Brazil and Mexico, obesity is no longer associated with relative wealth and is becoming a marker of poverty, as it is in developed countries.

People in the developing world are abandoning traditional diets that are rich in fibre and grain for diets that include increased levels of sugars, oils, and animal fats. This is partly due to changes in food processing and production, and partly to aggressive marketing techniques. In China, changes in diet, increased television viewing and reduced physical activity, all of which are linked to the process of urbanisation, have occurred in less than two decades. This is significant because it takes only 20 years for diabetes to become prevalent in populations who adopt a high-calorie, low activity lifestyle.

Many studies across the world have revealed that a person's ethnic heritage can affect his or her risk of developing diabetes. A recent study in America confirmed that Afrocaribbeans, Asians and Hispanics are more at risk, and that gaining weight may be a particularly strong diabetes risk factor for Asians. But it also had good news – that healthy eating habits may actually be more effective at lowering diabetes risk for these groups than for Caucasians.

One explanation for ethnic differences in diabetes risk is the 'thrifty gene' theory. This theory suggests that for some peoples adapted to a harsh environment, such as the Pima Indians of the Arizona desert, storing extra calories as fat was an evolutionary advantage as it would enable them to survive famines. Now, with changes in diet and activity levels, 70% of Pima Indians are obese and 50% of them have diabetes. Their thrifty gene, which was an asset to survival in the past, is a genetic liability in today's environment. A similar pattern can be seen amongst the peoples of the Pacific Islands.

Asians, and particularly Indians, may also have a 'thrifty gene'. India has the world's largest diabetic population, mostly in urban areas where as many as 12% of adults suffer from diabetes. Epidemiological studies have revealed that Indians are susceptible to diabetes, irrespective of the place they live in. Migrant Asian Indians living in different parts of the world are more likely to develop diabetes than other ethnic groups living in the same countries.

Causes of the Global Rise of Diabetes:

- **Increased global population**
- **Ageing population**
- **Urbanisation**
- **Obesogenic environment**
- **Increased dietary fat and sugar**
- **Reduced activity levels**
- **Ethnicity – the 'thrifty gene'**

While Caucasians may be at risk of diabetes if their Body Mass Index (BMI) is 30 and above, the risk for Indians, and for other Asians, increases at a BMI of 25 and above. The ideal body weight by international standards is below 25, but the ideal body mass index for an Indian appears to be below 23. Most diabetes occurs in the age group 50-60 for Caucasians, but an Indian is likely to get it younger – at around 45. Genetics also play a part: because diabetes runs in families, and because marriage between relatives is quite common in India, the genetic propensity to diabetes tends to be more strongly inherited.

The good news is that this predicted rise of diabetes is not inexorable. At the macro level, unhealthy dietary trends could be reversed by using public education, subsidising healthy foods and labelling foods clearly, but in practice it might be difficult to get global agreement on these issues. On an individual level, however, if people can change their dietary and lifestyle habits, some of which may have been acquired only quite recently, they can avoid diabetes before it arises, or live healthily with diabetes if they already have it.

Diabetes Self-Management

Whether you are on insulin, diabetes medication or just managing your diabetes through diet and weight control, there is a lot you can do to determine your own health status. Choosing foods that moderate glycaemic response, adopting an active lifestyle, monitoring your blood glucose, watching your weight, getting enough rest and avoiding stress are all part of responsible diabetes self-management.

Nutrition

Why is nutrition so important in diabetes? Well, it is without doubt the most important tool for keeping blood glucose levels under control. Other things may be responsible for upsetting blood glucose – for example infection or stress. But these are usually out of your control, whereas what you eat is entirely under your control, and it is a precise tool for doing the job. Many diabetics, particularly Type 1s who test their blood glucose frequently, know exactly which foods raise their blood glucose and by how much. Keeping blood glucose under tight control ensures that you are less likely to suffer the chronic complications of diabetes, so it makes sense to keep good nutrition at the centre of your diabetes management programme.

Diabetes UK say that the vast majority of newly-diagnosed diabetics who ring their help line have one overriding concern, and that is 'what can I eat?' The answer, in a nutshell, is a normal healthy diet. The key is the word 'healthy' – what does this really mean for most of us? I always advise my patients to eat foods as near to their natural state as possible, and if you do this you can't go wrong. By this I don't mean a raw food diet, but one in which each ingredient has been minimally processed, as would be the case in the diets of more primitive peoples. This applies to everybody, not just diabetics. That having been said, there are special considerations for people with diabetes. It has always seemed illogical to me to base a diet for people with diabetes on carbohydrates, as these are the foods that diabetics, by definition, have the most difficulty metabolising. A high intake of carbohydrates will inevitably lead to consistently high blood glucose levels in people who either don't have enough insulin or who are resistant to insulin.

The current recommendations from Diabetes UK and the American Diabetes Association, to base the diet on starchy carbohydrate foods such as bread, pasta, chapattis, potatoes, yam, noodles, rice and cereals, mean that you would be getting over 50% of your energy from carbohydrates, with 15% from protein sources and about 30% from fat. If this seems a lot of fat, note that these percentages refer to energy from each component, rather than volume of each component. Fat is a significant source of energy, but it doesn't take up much room.

A low fat, high carbohydrate diet, such as the current recommendations outlined above, in combination with regular exercise, is the traditional recommendation for treating diabetes. But in spite of a significant decrease in fat consumption and increase in carbohydrate consumption in the US and other developed countries over the last few decades, diabetes is still on the rise. It is well known that a high carbohydrate diet raises blood glucose after a meal, and therefore also raises insulin or insulin requirements. One of insulin's effects is to store fat, so more insulin leads to more fat storage. More fat storage leads to more insulin resistance, and a vicious cycle is set in motion. This apparent failure of the traditional diet for diabetes indicates that an alternative dietary approach is needed. Because carbohydrate is the major trigger for insulin production, some form of carbohydrate restriction seems to be the obvious answer. Evidence from various randomised controlled trials in recent years has convinced me that such diets are safe and effective. Most of these studies refer to Type 2, but studies also exist to prove that a lower carbohydrate diet works for Type 1 as well. One Swedish study put Type 1 patients on a diet limited to 70-90 g carbohydrates per day and taught them to match the insulin doses accordingly. The purpose was to reduce the blood glucose fluctuations and to improve HbA1c. And it worked –

The best diet for diabetes consists of:

- **Lots of vegetables**
- **Lots of pulses (lentils and beans)**
- **Moderate amount of fruit**
- **Moderate amount of whole grains, usually non-gluten grains**
- **Moderate amount of oily fish, nuts and seeds**
- **Small amount of poultry, red meat and low fat dairy products**
- **Very little or no processed foods, full fat dairy products, refined grains or sugars**

the patients' average HbA1c level was significantly reduced from 7.5 to 6.4 and remained lower for at least 12 months. Another long-term study of people with both Type 1 and Type 2 restricted the diet even further than the Swedish study – to 30 grams of carbohydrate per day. Again, the insulin-dependent patients were able to lower their insulin doses, in both groups the ratio between good and bad cholesterol improved, and the mean HbA1c scores decreased from 7.9 to 5.7.

The solution must surely be a lower carbohydrate diet, replacing carbohydrates with more protein and modest amounts of essential fats. I have therefore settled on a lower carbohydrate approach both with my patients and in this book, aiming for about 40% carbohydrate overall, with 30% fat and 30% protein. This is not difficult to achieve and doesn't involve a lot of deprivation. I am not advocating anything as radical as the Atkins diet, which contains far less carbohydrate, more protein and typically a high intake of saturated fat too, but it is useful to reflect that Dr Atkins originally formulated his high protein approach to help reduce insulin secretion, and thus fat storage, in people with Type 2 diabetes among others. One proviso is that if you are suffering from diabetic nephropathy or kidney disease, you should not increase your protein intake without consulting your doctor. Protein sometimes has to be restricted for people with kidney problems.

The diet I recommend is broadly similar to what is known as the Mediterranean diet. It is characterised by a high intake of vegetables, pulses, fruit and whole grains, and a low intake of red meat, processed meat, high-fat dairy products and refined grains. Protein comes mostly from oily fish, eggs, nuts, poultry, a little red meat, and pulses, carbohydrate comes largely from vegetables and some whole grains – usually non-gluten grains – and fat comes from oily fish, nuts, seeds and cold-pressed nut and seed oils.

How does this square with the numerous observations that diabetes risk increases for people in developing countries when they change from a traditional carbohydrate-rich diet to a more 'Western' diet? Are these 'Western' diets not higher in fat and protein, and if so why do they increase the diabetes risk when studies show that diets higher in fat and protein actually lower the risk? I think the answer lies not in diet alone. When people change to a more refined diet, it is as a result of urbanisation, so it is accompanied by an increasingly sedentary lifestyle. If you simply turn on a tap instead of having to walk several miles a day to collect water, or open a packet of flour instead of vigorously pounding grain, then you cannot afford to eat as much carbohydrate because your energy output is much lower. And if that flour is refined instead of wholegrain, and if you use refined polyunsaturated oils instead of natural oils like coconut oil, then these factors will increase your diabetes risk.

Carbohydrate Foods

The Glycaemic Index and Glycaemic Load

The Glycaemic Index and Glycaemic Load have been widely publicised in recent years, and most people are now familiar with these terms. The Glycaemic Index was first formulated in the 1980s, when scientists conducted a series of trials in which volunteers were given a single food to eat after a fast of some hours. The rise in their blood glucose was then measured over four hours to see the glycaemic effect of each food. They found that all carbohydrates, regardless of whether they were thought to be 'simple' or 'complex', cause a peak in blood glucose approximately 30 minutes after being eaten. Secondly, they found that some carbohydrates cause a much more dramatic rise than others.

Glucose was given a value of 100, and all other carbohydrates were ranked according to their effect on blood glucose levels. This ranking is known as the Glycaemic Index (GI). Carbohydrates that cause a sharp rise in blood glucose have the highest GI, whereas carbohydrates that have a gentler effect on blood glucose have a low GI. There are several factors that affect the GI of a food. The first is the proportion of carbohydrate in relation to protein and fat. Neither protein nor fat affect blood glucose at all, so the lower the proportion of carbohydrate in a food, the lower the GI and the lower the glycaemic response will be. Secondly, the gelatinisation of a starchy carbohydrate has an effect on its GI. If pasta is cooked until it is soft, the starch has had more time to absorb water, and consequently is more gelatinous than if the pasta is cooked 'al dente'. So the well-cooked pasta will have a higher GI than 'al dente' pasta. Cooking generally has this effect, especially on root vegetables. For example, cooked carrots have a higher GI than raw carrots. Viscous, soluble fibres such as rolled oats, beans and lentils increase the viscosity of the contents of the intestine and this slows down the interaction between the starch and the enzymes which break it down. This results in a lower GI than, say, less viscous fibre such as wheat flour. Similarly, if a food consists of small particles, for example white flour, it is easier for water and digestive enzymes to penetrate the particles, and consequently glucose from white flour will hit the bloodstream sooner than that from the large particles in stone-ground flour, so white flour has a higher GI. And finally, acid in foods slows down stomach emptying, thereby slowing the rate at which the starch can be digested. This effect can be seen by adding vinegar or lemon juice to a food.

But the Glycaemic Index on its own is not a very effective tool for assessing the glycaemic effect of a meal. For example, it is useful to know that raisins have a high GI, as this would warn you not to eat too many raisins, or at least not on their own. But this does not mean you have to avoid raisins, just that you should eat them in moderation, and combined with protein and fat, such as for example in a curry.

The Glycemic Load was formulated to measure the total glycaemic response to a food or to a meal. The GL is equivalent to the GI value of a food multiplied by the amount of carbohydrate per serving and divided by 100. A meal contains a variety of different foods, so how do you work out the GI or GL value of a whole meal? Briefly, this is done by adding up all the grams of carbohydrate in the meal, working out what percentage each food contributes to the total carbohydrate content, and then multiplying this percentage by the GI value. A food with a GL of 20 or more is high, a GL of 11 to 19 inclusive is medium, and a GL of 10 or less is low.

An exact calculation is difficult and at times impossible, because the GI and GL of all foods have not yet been measured. I have therefore adopted a traffic light system for the recipes in this book, stating whether the GL is low, medium or high, and giving the percentage of carbohydrate. The lists at the back of this book give both GI and GL values for reference. I have used the latest tables available, those published in the *American Journal of Clinical Nutrition* in 2002. These tables often give the results of several different studies for the same food. For example, there are 10 studies on bananas, giving a GI anywhere between 30 and 58, and a GL between 6 (for a Danish study on underripe bananas) to 16 (for a South African study on ripe bananas). For this reason, I have not attempted to give an exact GL for each

A list of proven diabetic-friendly foods:
- **Vegetables, especially onions & garlic, the cabbage family, beetroot, celery, courgettes, radishes and tomatoes**
- **Fruit, especially apples, berries, cherries, grapefruit and plums**
- **Wholegrains especially buckwheat, brown basmati rice, quinoa and pearl barley**
- **Pulses, especially mung beans, beansprouts and soya products**
- **Oily fish, almonds and coconut oil**
- **Green tea**
- **Spices, especially cinnamon and turmeric**

recipe, and my 'traffic lights' are for guidance only. For example, the Scottish groats on page 31 are fairly high GL. This means that you should plan to eat a protein food at the same meal, such as a boiled egg or a piece of fish. It does not mean that you should avoid oat groats, which have some very desirable qualities. To further complicate things, some diabetics tell me that oat porridge gives them a glucose spike, whereas others swear it's the best breakfast for keeping their blood glucose steady. Personal experience is the best guide in this case.

The Glycaemic Index and Glycaemic Load were never intended to be used in isolation. A food can have a low GI but still be high in saturated fat or have other undesirable qualities. For example a Mars Bar has a moderate GI of about 65 because the effect of the glucose is moderated by the presence of partially hydrogenated soybean oil, condensed milk and cocoa butter, so it is hardly a healthy choice.

Although carbohydrates should be limited, they should definitely not be avoided completely, because they are an important source of energy. But it is important to choose the right sort of carbohydrates – vegetables, fruit, wholegrains and pulses. Bear in mind that some of these foods have a greater carbohydrate percentage than others. Grains have the most, followed by fruit and vegetables. There are trace amounts of protein and essential fats in many vegetables, which shouldn't be underestimated, especially in a vegetarian diet. Beans are a fairly balanced combination of carbohydrate and protein.

Vegetables

It is important to eat a wide variety of vegetables. They are rich in fibre and nutrients and help to protect the cardiovascular system and nerves from glycosylation. Avoid cooked starchy root vegetables especially potatoes and parsnips as they have a very high GI value. New potatoes are the exception, as they have a moderate GI.

Certain vegetables are particularly beneficial, such as onions and garlic, as they contain active ingredients that appear to increase insulin in the blood by preventing it being inactivated by the liver. Beetroot, broccoli, celery, cabbage, chicory, Chinese cabbage, courgettes, kale, radishes and tomatoes are also reputed to have antidiabetic effects.

Raw vegetables and vegetable juices are especially valuable. Vegetable juices are an excellent source of vitamins and minerals and other phyto-nutrients that have been shown to combat disease. Because juices are raw, the vitamin C and other water-soluble vitamins and enzymes that would be lost in cooking are still intact. Juices are easily absorbed and therefore offer instant energy without pushing up the blood glucose. The juice of sweeter vegetables, such as carrot and beetroot, should be treated with caution and only drunk mixed with that of green leafy vegetables such as spinach or watercress to mitigate any possible rise in blood glucose.

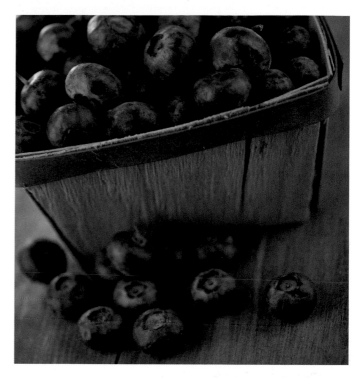

Fruit

Choose low GI fruits such as apples, pears, cherries and plums. Berries are also a good choice owing to their high antioxidant content, for example blueberries, raspberries and strawberries. High GI fruits such as melon and bananas should be eaten sparingly. Grapefruit, which has a very low GI, may be one of the healthiest dietary choices for people with diabetes and for those trying to lose weight, because it contains enzymes that help control insulin spikes that occur after a meal, thus freeing the digestive system to process food more efficiently, with the result that fewer nutrients are stored as fat.

Consumption of all fruit should be fairly moderate, as fruit is a significant source of fructose (fruit sugar). Dried fruits, because they have had most of their moisture removed, tend to be high GI and should be used in only small amounts. Dried apricots, however, have a moderate GI of about 44.

It is wise to avoid fruit juice, or to dilute it with water. Most fruit juice provides about 10 grams of sugar per 100 grams –

about the same as a cola drink. In fact, orange juice is used by many insulin-dependent diabetics after a hypo precisely because it raises blood glucose so rapidly.

Wholegrains

Wholegrains, the outer husk of which has not been removed by processing, are a good source of unrefined carbohydrate, but they should be eaten in moderate portions only.

One of the most beneficial grains for people with diabetes is buckwheat, which is readily available in health food shops. It is not related to wheat so it's gluten-free, and is not even technically a grain but a seed. Several studies have shown than buckwheat may help increase insulin sensitivity through the action of a component called chiro-inositol which may prompt cells to become more receptive to insulin. Chiro-inositol is relatively high in buckwheat and rarely found in other foods. There are a couple of small studies published in China and India indicating that people with Type 2 diabetes who consumed buckwheat had better glycaemic control. The GI of buckwheat has been extensively tested and is about 54, and its glycaemic load is 16, which is medium.

In the recipes I have used buckwheat, brown basmati rice, pearl barley and quinoa, as these all have a low GI value. Whole grains contain chromium, needed for carbohydrate metabolism, and lots of minerals and vitamins. Avoid any products made with refined white flour. Not only is it high GI, but it is almost devoid of nutritional value.

Because there is a link between Type 1 diabetes and celiac disease, many diabetics have to avoid the gluten grains (wheat, barley, rye and commercially grown oats). Most of the grains I use in these recipes are gluten-free (brown rice, quinoa, buckwheat, corn). Where I have used gluten grains, I have suggested gluten-free substitutes where suitable. For thickening sauces and making cakes I always use gluten-free flour as a matter of course.

I have only included two bread recipes – one for spelt bread, because it has a moderate GI of 63 and because some people intolerant to wheat can tolerate spelt – and the other for rolls that contain lentils which help to offset the high glycaemic effect of wheat flour. Bread should not really be used as a staple by people with diabetes owing to its high carbohydrate content. If you cannot do without bread, try wholegrain pumpernickel or Burgen Soy Lin bread as it has the lowest GI of any bread ever tested.

Beans and Pulses

Beans and pulses are admirably well-balanced foods. They are a good source of protein, complex carbohydrates, fibre and minerals, are low in fat, and generally have a very low GI. Sprouting beans makes them particularly nutritious, as sprouts are full of enzymes. Mung beans, usually eaten as beansprouts, have been found to be helpful as an antidiabetic, low GI food, rich in antioxidants.

Soya products, such as soya beans, tofu, miso and tempeh are excellent sources of vegetable protein. Soya protein can have a positive effect on blood fats and on kidney function in diabetic patients, and can decrease LDL, the 'bad' cholesterol, by as much as 10-20%. Introduce beans into your diet gently, as they can be hard to digest if you're not used to them. Adding a piece of root ginger or a strip of kombu seaweed to the boiling water seems to help make beans more digestible.

Protein Foods

Amino acids, the breakdown products of protein foods, are normally referred to as the 'building blocks' of the body, in that their primary role is maintenance and repair. But our bodies will also use protein to make glucose. Since glucose, usually made from carbohydrates, is what gives us energy, it is important for a person with diabetes who is limiting their carbohydrates to eat enough protein. (People with renal failure, however, may be advised to limit protein). Protein has the effect of slowing the absorption of glucose from carbohydrates, so always make sure you eat a small portion of protein at each snack or meal. Choose fish, especially the oily fish such as organic or wild salmon and mackerel, eggs, live natural yoghurt, cottage cheese, pulses, quinoa, soya and poultry.

It may be wise to limit the amount of red meat you eat if you have diabetes. A study has indicated that the consumption of red meat, which contains haem iron, is associated with an increased risk of Type 2 diabetes, and I mentioned above that Type 1 diabetes could be associated with increased meat consumption. I have included a couple of recipes in this book for lamb, which is generally a better choice than beef or pork because sheep are more likely to have been raised naturally and fed on grass. There is no doubt that meat is a good source of protein, zinc and B vitamins, so eating it occasionally and in small amounts is fine.

Dairy Products

Milk is a controversial topic in nutrition circles. It is a whole food, containing protein, fats and carbohydrate, but a whole food for calves, not necessarily for humans. The protein fraction, casein, can be a problem for many people, and most of the world's adult population lacks the enzyme necessary to digest lactose (milk sugar). In fact, the ability to digest lactose after the age of 4 or 5 is seen by some researchers as a genetic mutation, found only in people of Western European descent.

We know that dairy products are associated with the development of Type 1 diabetes in some children, which may be a good argument for not giving cow's milk to babies and children who have Type 1 diabetes in their families, but does this mean that people with established diabetes should avoid dairy products? Well, yes and no. I think you should probably avoid cow's milk, but not necessarily all dairy products.

There were two recent pieces of research linking the consumption of cow's milk to increasing levels of obesity, diabetes and heart disease. The British Women's Heart and Health Study looked at over 4,000 older women and found that those who avoided milk were half as likely to have metabolic syndrome as milk drinkers. The second study looked at the diets and weights of nearly 13,000 children over a period of three years. Those children consuming more than three servings of (low-fat) milk per day were approximately 35% more likely to become overweight than those who drank just one or two glasses. This may be because dairy products cause an unusual increase in insulin secretion, which as we have seen encourages fat deposition.

Milk is not even a good source of calcium, as is often claimed, because it does not contain enough magnesium to balance the calcium. These two minerals are mutually dependent in the body, each requiring the other for absorption, so foods which are already calcium/magnesium balanced, such as seeds, nuts, dark green leafy vegetables and wholegrains, are really preferable to milk.

In cultures where the population lacks lactase, fermented dairy products such as yoghurt are commonly eaten because the bacteria in live yoghurt predigest the lactose in the milk. I use a lot of yoghurt in cooking and have provided a recipe for making your own yoghurt, labneh (a yoghurt cheese) and paneer (Indian soft cheese). Butter is acceptable in small amounts as it is nearly all fat and contains virtually no protein. I do use butter in baking and in recipes where the taste of the fat is important, and I also use feta and other goat's cheeses in moderation.

Fats and Oils

Fat does not increase blood glucose levels, but that does not mean that fats can be eaten indiscriminately, for there are good fats and bad fats. It is very important to avoid scrupulously any trans-fatty acids or hydrogenated fats (most cooking fats, margarines and processed foods) and refined oils. A large, long-term study of 84,000 women recently found that trans-fatty acids can raise a woman's risk of Type 2 diabetes, while substituting foods rich in trans fats with those that contain polyunsaturated fats could reduce the risk by about 40%.

The mono-unsaturated fats, such as extra virgin olive oil, and the omega-3 fatty acids found in oily fish and nuts, actually lower blood fats and contribute to glycaemic control in people with diabetes. Avocados and olives are good sources of monounsaturated fatty acids and tasty additions to the diet.

There are only three fats and oils that I recommend for cooking – extra virgin olive oil, virgin coconut oil and organic butter, with occasional use of groundnut oil for high temperature stir frying as it has a high burning point. For salad dressings, extra virgin olive oil or any of the cold-pressed seed or nut oils may be used, such as walnut oil and flax seed oil (rich in Omega 3 fatty acids), avocado oil or pumpkin seed oil. For spreading, try almond or hazelnut butter or tahini (sesame seed paste). Organic butter is also an acceptable choice, as it is a rich source of fat-soluble vitamins, trace minerals and medium chain fatty acids (MCFA) which are a good energy source.

Coconut oil has some interesting properties that make it very suitable for people with diabetes. It helps to regulate blood glucose, thus lessening the effects of diabetes. It also raises the metabolic rate causing the body to burn up more calories and thus promoting weight loss. A faster metabolic rate stimulates increased production of needed insulin and increases absorption of glucose into cells, thus helping both

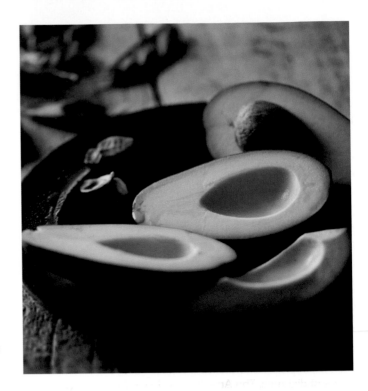

Type 1 and Type 2 diabetics. Coconut oil is composed of about 50% lauric acid. Like other MCFAs, lauric acid is digested and processed differently from other fats. It is sent directly to the liver where it is immediately converted into energy – just like a carbohydrate. Numerous studies have shown that replacing long chain fatty acids with MCFAs results in a decrease in body weight gain and a reduction in fat deposition. Furthermore, reports from India reveal that Type 2 diabetes there has increased as people have abandoned coconut oil in favour of refined vegetable oils. Organic coconut oil is available from Higher Nature (see Useful Addresses).

Nuts and Seeds

Nuts and seeds are nutrient-dense and contain essential fats, protein and some fibre. The best nuts are those with a higher proportion of monounsaturated fatty acids, such as macadamia nuts, hazelnuts, pecans and almonds. Almonds are particularly important for people with diabetes. A recent study found that supplementing the diet with almonds not only helped people to lose weight but also enabled Type 1 diabetics to reduce their medication. Nuts such as almonds and seeds are rich in magnesium, a mineral in which most diabetics are deficient. It is therefore important to increase consumption of major food sources of magnesium, such as whole grains, nuts, and green leafy vegetables. Nuts and seeds can be eaten as a snack with a piece of fruit, or ground and added to porridge, live yoghurt or vegetable juices to increase fibre intake. Avoid salted or dry roasted nuts.

Sugar and Other Sweeteners

Sugar consumption and the incidence of diabetes appear to have kept pace with each other in the developing world. However, there is no proof that eating sugar is the direct cause of diabetes. The American Diabetes Association (ADA) no longer advises people with diabetes to avoid sugar. However, since they are sponsored by Cadbury-Schweppes, the world's largest manufacturer of sweets, their advice may not be impartial. Similarly, Diabetes UK no longer forbids sugar. However, there are plenty of reasons why diabetics, along with everyone else, should avoid it. Reducing the amount of sugar in the diet helps to reduce weight which in turn improves glycaemic control.

White sugar is particularly damaging as the B vitamins and trace minerals such as zinc, manganese, chromium, selenium and cobalt are all removed by the refining process. As these substances are necessary for the body to metabolise sugar, the sugar squanders these nutrients from the body's reserves. Sugar also suppresses the immune system and has a hand in numerous other conditions, such as elevated cholesterol, kidney damage, depression, hormonal imbalance, free radical formation, hypertension, migraines and osteoporosis.

Fructose is the form of sugar found in fruit, as its name suggests. The consumption of refined fructose, primarily from high-fructose corn syrup (HFCS), has increased considerably in the United States and across the world during the past several decades. Some nutritionists believe fructose is a safer form of sugar than sucrose, particularly for people with diabetes, because it does not adversely affect blood glucose regulation, at least in the short-term. It has a GI of about 19, much lower than that of sugar. However, refined fructose has potentially harmful effects on other aspects of metabolism. In particular, it seems to encourage the formation of toxic advanced glycation end-products (TAGEs), which play a role in the development of diabetes complications and atherosclerosis. Fructose has also been implicated as the main cause of symptoms in some patients with irritable bowel syndrome. Of particular concern for diabetics, fructose appears to reduce the sensitivity of insulin receptors and raise blood fats significantly. It is metabolised by the liver and converts to fat more easily than any other sugar, which explains why some researchers think that fructose may be responsible in part for the increasing prevalence of obesity. When naturally contained within fruits and vegetables, where it is in small quantities and accompanied by dietary fibre, fructose causes no problems, so people should not be discouraged from eating these healthy foods.

A new natural sugar on the market is agave nectar which is 90% fructose. This honey-like liquid derived from the agave cactus is 25% sweeter than sugar, with a GI of 11 and a GL of only 1. It performs well in cooking, but in view of its cost and the high fructose content, I can't recommend it.

Unfortunately people with diabetes are often encouraged to replace sugar with substances that could be even more harmful in the long run – sweeteners. These should be avoided because they promote a sweet tooth and increase cravings for sweet foods, thus making it more difficult to lose weight. A possible explanation is that when you eat an artificial sweetener, the body prepares itself to digest carbohydrates which then fail to materialise. When you do subsequently eat

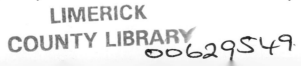

some carbohydrate the body compromises by creating a greater than normal rise in blood glucose. Not only that, but some sweeteners may have more sinister drawbacks. **Aspartame**, an odourless powder 200 times sweeter than sugar, is processed using methanol which is highly toxic. Complaints about its effects range from headaches to seizures, although these are not substantiated. It is marketed as Canderel in the UK and Nutrasweet in the USA. **Sucralose**, which is marketed as Splenda, has no calories and is about 600 times sweeter than sugar. It is produced by chlorinating sugar. Studies have shown that it has no effect on blood glucose in diabetics, but it has been reported to cause migraines in some people.

There are three forms of natural sweetener on the market that are safer than the artificial sweeteners but have their own drawbacks. The first is FOS, (**Fructo-oligosaccharides**), obtainable from health food shops. FOS can be used in baking and to sweeten stewed fruit. It is mildly sweet and nourishes the beneficial bacteria in the gut. However, it can cause flatulence and bloating and some people find it unpleasant to use for this reason. The second is **Stevia**, a natural plant sweetener from a member of the chrysanthemum family. Stevia is banned in the EU and the USA as a foodstuff because of fears it may produce adverse effects in the male reproductive system and damage DNA. Many diabetics do use it in spite of these concerns, and in spite of its unpleasant aftertaste. Finally there is a naturally occurring sugar substitute called **Xylitol** that is crystalline in form and looks and tastes like sugar but with 40% less calories. It is a popular sugar substitute for people with diabetes as it has a low GI (7) and therefore has little effect on blood glucose levels. The main side-effect of xylitol is mild diarrhoea in people who use it in large quantities. A side issue is that it is toxic to dogs. When I was experimenting with it for this book my dog ate a whole packet (250 grams) and nearly died of acute hypoglycaemia, so I am a little prejudiced against it.

I still think that the best approach to sugar and sweeteners is to use only natural sweeteners in as small quantities as possible (bearing in mind that these are still concentrated forms of sugar) whilst trying to re-educate your palate, so that you do not crave sweet foods. Fruit, especially dried fruit, can fulfil the need for sweetness without the health concerns attached to artificial sweeteners or concentrated sweeteners such as fructose or stevia. In the recipes I use only organic brown sugar, honey and concentrated apple juice.

According to relatively new findings, honey may have some significant health effects. In addition to its primary carbohydrate content, honey often contains polyphenols, which can act as antioxidants. As a nutritional element, antioxidants prevent oxidative stress to cells throughout the body. Furthermore, honey has been shown to be effective in increasing the populations of probiotic bacteria in the gut, which may help strengthen the immune system, improve digestion, lower cholesterol and prevent colon cancer.

Drinks

Caffeine drinks

Controversy rages in the scientific community about the effects of caffeine on diabetes risk and glucose control.

Coffee

It is known that drinking large amounts of coffee or drinks containing caffeine can increase blood pressure in people who do not normally drink coffee. Interestingly, this does not happen in habitual coffee drinkers. In fact, no clear association between coffee and the risk of hypertension, heart attack, or other cardiovascular diseases has been demonstrated. In contrast to early studies, recent research indicates that habitual moderate coffee intake does not represent a health hazard and may even be associated with beneficial effects on cardiovascular health. Several epidemiological studies over the past few years have concluded that drinking coffee can reduce the risk of diabetes. A 20 year Finnish study found that drinking coffee was associated with lower heart disease and lower death rate in diabetics. The Atherosclerosis Risk In Communities (ARIC) Study in the USA found that increased coffee consumption was significantly associated with a decreased risk of Type 2 diabetes. The Iowa Women's Health Study of 29,000 women over 9 years found the same relationship, especially if the coffee was decaffeinated. A similar large study, the Nurses' Health Study II, found that moderate consumption of both caffeinated and decaffeinated coffee may lower risk of Type 2 diabetes and suggested that coffee constituents other than caffeine, such as chlorogenic acid and quinides, may be responsible. However, coffee has other disadvantages, as it may interfere with your body's ability to keep homocysteine and cholesterol levels in check, probably by inhibiting the action of the vitamins folate, B12 or B6, but the majority of research clearly shows that 1-2 cups per day cause no harm and may even be advantageous.

Tea

Black tea has been observed to reduce blood glucose in Type 2 diabetes in animal studies, and to protect against heart disease in humans, though a small German study recently found that putting milk in tea blocks the effect of catechins, the flavonoids in tea responsible for its benefits to the heart and cardiovascular system.

Japanese studies of green tea, which is drunk without milk, have found it to be protective against diabetes, especially in women, although other studies have found no clear effects of daily green tea consumption on blood glucose level, HbA1c level, insulin resistance or inflammation markers. However, it is known that the polyphenols in green tea have antioxidant and anti-inflammatory properties and are therefore heart-protective.

Fizzy drinks

Fizzy drinks and cordials should be avoided as they are high in sugar. Diet drinks contain sweeteners such as aspartame and should also be avoided. This also applies to the currently fashionable flavoured waters. A recent American study found that in adults with diabetes who had one or more drinks of diet soda per day, their HbA1c level was 0.7 units greater compared to those who drank none. Instead of fizzy drinks, choose water, vegetable juices, highly diluted fruit juices, herbal teas, water, dandelion coffee, green tea, or hot water with lemon or ginger.

Alcohol

Moderate alcohol consumption, as opposed to total abstinence, seems to be associated with a decreased incidence of heart disease in people with diabetes, according to a recent review of the scientific literature on the subject. A French study has found that insulin resistance is low in people with regular mild to moderate alcohol consumption but higher in both heavy drinkers and people who don't drink alcohol at all. Moderate alcohol consumption means two or three units of alcohol per day. However, some people should not consume alcohol because of the medication they take for diabetes or other conditions.

The dangers of heavy drinking, on the other hand, are even more acute for people with diabetes than for anyone else. They include hypoglycaemia, glucose intolerance, and ketone and lactate accumulation. The growing alcohol consumption in young people, particularly in young women, may be a risk factor for the development of Type 2 diabetes.

Sports drinks

Sports drinks usually contain water, sugar and electrolytes. These drinks are not really necessary for most people and they can cause blood glucose levels to rise too high in people with diabetes. Whilst it is important to replace lost fluids you do not necessarily need to buy special sports drinks – water will work just as well.

Convenience Foods

Convenience foods and ready meals should be avoided whenever possible. Read labels carefully to check for saturated fat, fibre and sugar content. Hidden sugars include corn syrup, dextrose and fructose. Low fat foods are often higher in sugar.

Diabetic Products

I do not recommend the purchase or consumption of special diabetic products. Foods that are labelled 'diabetic' aren't necessarily healthier or more suitable for diabetics than other foods, and tend to be more expensive than other products. Many of the products that are labelled 'diabetic' are sweets, chocolates and biscuits. We should all avoid eating lots of these types of foods.

Salt

It is well-known that salt should be used very sparingly by anyone with high blood pressure, and that applies to many people with diabetes. However, blood pressure depends not just on the amount of sodium in the body, but also on the amount of potassium, found in abundance in fruit and vegetables. As always, balance is the key. I think that if your diet is high in fruit and vegetables, you can afford to use a little salt in your cooking, provided it is sea salt which contains some trace minerals. You should, however, avoid processed foods which are high in salt, or adding extra salt at the table.

Herbs and Spices

Several culinary herbs have been shown to help improve the action of insulin in lowering blood glucose levels. These include coriander, bay, juniper berries, fenugreek seed, cloves, turmeric, and cinnamon, and you will find many uses for these spices in the recipes that follow. Cinnamon is thought to be

particularly effective and is widely used in the Indian traditional system of medicine to treat diabetes. A 2003 study found that just 1g (less than half a teaspoon) of cinnamon per day reduced blood glucose levels by 20% in people with Type 2 diabetes, as well as cholesterol and other blood fats. A recent study identified the active agent as cinnamaldehyde, which appears to reduce blood glucose and HbA1c. Cinnamon contains both fat-soluble and water-soluble fractions and there is some evidence that high levels of the fat-soluble fractions of cinnamon could be cause for concern if a person is taking 1g per day. One solution is to make an infusion of cinnamon by boiling it in water, then straining the liquid through muslin and discarding the pulp. The liquid, which will contain only the water-soluble fraction, can then be drunk as a tea or used in food.

Vitamins and Minerals

As a nutritional therapist I believe that even those who think they eat a well balanced diet are not getting the ideal intake of vitamins and minerals. And people suffering from a chronic disease such as diabetes are at greater need of these vitamins and minerals than the rest of the population. Diabetics are under more oxidative stress than other people, so they need more antioxidants. As chronic inflammation is part of the picture, a higher intake of anti-inflammatory essential fats is necessary. Glucose metabolism is impaired in diabetes, so the nutrient co-factors for glucose metabolism are needed in higher amounts, and retention and absorption of certain minerals are compromised in diabetes. I have taken this into account in the recipes, and the nutritional notes that accompany each recipe should alert you to which foods are particularly good sources of these nutrients. However, I do believe that nutritional supplementation is necessary for diabetics and would advise anyone reading this book to work with a nutritional therapist in consultation with their diabetes care team to determine the right balance of supplements.

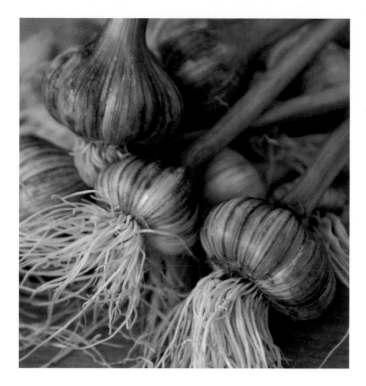

Magnesium is probably the single most important mineral as it is involved in glucose metabolism, is a component of many different enzyme systems in the body, and is often found to be deficient in people with diabetes. It helps to transport glucose across cell membranes. Scientists believe that a deficiency of magnesium interrupts insulin secretion in the pancreas and increases insulin resistance in the body's tissues. Magnesium deficiency appears to be common among people with diabetes, and such a deficiency appears to worsen the blood glucose control in Type 2 diabetes. The best food sources of magnesium are quinoa, beans and pulses, muesli, Brazil nuts and whole wheat.

Chromium is one of the major components of glucose tolerance factor, a molecule that improves the ability of insulin to lower blood glucose levels. In fact, without adequate chromium, insulin cannot be activated and blood glucose goes out of control. Chromium is found in brewers yeast, wholemeal bread, rye bread, oysters, potatoes and wheat germ, with traces in beetroot and onions.

Zinc is another mineral needed for glucose metabolism and is also important for immunity. It is found in oysters, popcorn, sesame seeds, pumpkin seeds, crab, lobster and walnuts.

Selenium is an important antioxidant and there's very little of it in the soil these days, so consumption of Brazil nuts is helpful, as each nut contains the recommended daily allowance of selenium. It is also found in molasses, clams, cashews and white fish.

Of the vitamins, the B vitamins are very important as they are needed for glucose metabolism and for the energy cycle. Some of them (vitamins B2, B6, folic acid and B12) are needed to deactivate the toxic by product of protein metabolism – homocysteine. If the diet is short of certain B vitamins, the body fails to detoxify homocysteine, and levels therefore increase. These increased levels of homocysteine are linked to cardiovascular disease risk. Good sources of B vitamins are rice bran, beef and lamb's liver, peanuts, muesli and brewer's yeast.

Vitamin C is an important antioxidant. Humans cannot make vitamin C and therefore need to get it from their diet. Its virtues are too numerous to mention, but of particular interest to diabetics is its ability to reduce levels of C-reactive protein (CRP), an indicator of chronic inflammation, thought to be linked to increased risk of heart disease and diabetes. Vitamin C is found in all fruits and vegetables, but the richest sources are guavas, Brussels sprouts (raw), raw peppers, blackcurrants and kiwi fruit.

Vitamin E is a fat-soluble antioxidant found in wheat germ oil, soybean oil, almonds, sunflower seed oil and walnuts. Vitamin E works by protecting fats in the body from oxidation. It reduces LDL cholesterol, helps to improve blood flow to the retina, and protects nerve function.

Vitamins C and E seem to work together. Vitamin C helps to recycle vitamin E, and they appear to have a synergistic effect in protecting against diabetic nephropathy.

Finally, vitamin D may be an important vitamin in diabetes, as a deficiency of this vitamin has been associated with insulin deficiency and insulin resistance. Vitamin D is made in the body by exposure to sunshine, and is also found in mackerel, herring, kippers, salmon and sardines.

Snacks

Snacks are a very important tool for people with diabetes, though less so for those who are using a combination of long-acting and fast-acting insulin, or who are lucky enough to have an insulin pump. For those who are less able to keep their blood glucose levels steady, snacks should be consumed between meals. But they have to be balanced snacks (see page 47). A snack consisting solely of carbohydrate will have a marked effect on blood glucose, whereas a combination of protein and a low GI carbohydrate will keep the blood glucose more even. An exception is when people with diabetes, usually Type 1, experience a hypoglycaemic episode (a 'hypo'), when their blood glucose level dips below 70mg/dl and they feel shaky and weak, or perhaps start talking incoherently. Then they need a high GI carbohydrate snack, and they need it fast, or they are in danger of passing out. Most diabetics have their own personal choice of high glucose food to raise their blood glucose quickly. Some people use pure glucose tablets, some use orange juice or sugar lumps.

Eating Out

If you are insulin-dependent or take diabetes medication, you may need to think about when you will eat as well as what you will eat when you go to a restaurant. Try to eat at your usual time if possible. If that is not possible, eat a snack beforehand to keep your blood glucose level steady.

Trying out different cuisines is one of the pleasures of life, and there is no need for people with diabetes to avoid any particular style of restaurant. It's just wise to observe a few simple rules. Avoid fatty and salty snacks before the meal – choose vegetable crudités or olives where they are available. For starters, go for vegetable soups, salads or seafood rather than fried foods. For your main course, go for plain grilled fish, chicken or meat with lots of vegetables or salad. Avoid creamy sauces and dressings, and eat only small portions of pastry, white rice, potatoes and pasta. For dessert choose fresh fruit if it is available, fruit based desserts, or cheese and fruit without the biscuits.

Indian restaurants should offer lots of opportunities for diabetes-friendly eating, but unfortunately curries are too often swimming in oil and sometimes cream as well. Opt for plain kebabs, tandoori dishes, dhal, fish, raitas, most chutneys, plain poppadums and small portions only of plain boiled basmati rice. Sadly, brown rice is rarely served in Indian restaurants. Skip the desserts which tend to be very sweet indeed.

Chinese food is usually a healthy choice; though take care to avoid dishes that are deep fried or high in fat and sodium, especially in the sauces. Opt for steamed fish with ginger, steamed or stir fried vegetables, bean curd, plain chicken or shrimp dishes without batter and plain steamed rice. But beware – if you do find yourself eating very large amounts of 'safe' foods such as beansprouts, bok choy, mushrooms, bamboo shoots, you risk suffering from what Dr Bernstein calls 'the Chinese restaurant effect'. This can occur if you stuff yourself with low carbohydrate foods. The pancreas releases both insulin and glucagon when you eat carbohydrates, even low GI carbohydrates, to enable it to fine-tune the glycaemic response, but if you're deficient in insulin, as diabetics are, there may be too much glucagon, which will send your blood glucose too high. The moral is, therefore, never overeat, even in Chinese restaurants.

Thai food is a good choice for diabetics. Choose clear hot and sour soups, satay, fish cakes, stir fried chicken and seafood, curries and coconut dishes with a little boiled rice, but avoid anything deep fried.

The idea of Italian food, in most people's minds, may be synonymous with pasta and pizza, which you should avoid or only eat in modest amounts, as they are both made with refined white flour, but there are many other options to choose from. Italians have many wonderful ways with vegetable dishes and salads, so explore these when you can, or choose plain grilled fish or meat.

In Greek, Turkish and Lebanese restaurants, it is easy to choose grilled kebabs or fish. Meze, the typical hors d'oeuvres, offer options such as hummus, tzatziki, salads with feta cheese and olives, all of which are good choices. Avoid deep fried starters such as falafel.

Shopping

There is a suggested shopping list at the back of this book to help you make healthy choices when you are out shopping. I live in rural mid-Wales, and have been able to source locally every ingredient I use in this book. You should be able to get most of the ingredients in a big supermarket, but you will find fresher fruit and vegetables if you can shop in farmers markets and local greengrocers. For more exotic produce, try Asian markets which often stock items for their local population that are unavailable in supermarkets. Health food shops are a good hunting ground for more unusual grains, cereals, beans, nuts and seeds, often at better prices than in the supermarkets; and the advent of internet shopping has made availability of unusual ingredients even easier.

The largest proportion of items in your shopping basket should be fresh vegetables, but frozen vegetables are a good second choice. The rest should consist of fresh or frozen fruit, or fruit tinned in its own juice, whole grains, dried or tinned pulses, fish, eggs, a little lean meat and low fat dairy products. You can get help on what to shop for by visiting the virtual supermarket at Diabetes UK's Store Tour (www.storetour.co.uk). As you negotiate your way through the aisles of the virtual store tour choosing products, you are provided with nutritional information on each food or drink product and advice and feedback on your final shopping basket selections. Some supermarkets run similar store tours led by dieticians, so it is worth asking your local supermarket if these are available in your area.

Cooking Notes

I don't use any special equipment, except for a food processor, which I find invaluable for blending and mixing. You will find that I frequently recommend using the food processor to make purées and soups, or for fine chopping. If you don't have a food processor, you can usually make do with a blender, pestle and mortar, hand-cranked food mill or a sharp knife and some elbow grease.

If you are using a fan oven, reduce the temperature by 20°C.

Most recipes serve 4 people unless otherwise stated.

I have not given the sodium content of any dish, because most recipes specify adding salt 'to taste'. If you are trying to cut down on sodium, it is up to you to use as little salt as you can.

I have added a margin note if the recipe is naturally high in sodium. Note that sodium occurs naturally in celery, seafood, olives and kelp.

Quantities of ingredients are given in metric/imperial and in US measures. I recommend that you stick with one system of measurement, as measurements do vary. For example, the American tablespoon of a solid ingredient is a level spoon, whereas English tablespoons of solid ingredients are usually rounded, so that 1 English tablespoon equals about 1 1/2 American tablespoons.

breakfasts

pumpkin seed
and almond muesli

Makes approx. 20 servings **Time taken:** 10 minutes

450g/1lb (6 cups) Jumbo oat flakes
225g/8 oz (3 cups) Oat bran
110g/4 oz (³/4 cup) Pumpkin seeds
110g/4 oz (³/4 cup) Sunflower seeds
225g/8 oz (1³/4 cups) Natural almonds, sliced
Water, apple juice or milk for soaking
Optional, to serve: Dried or fresh fruit of your choice
Natural live yoghurt (see page 140) or soya yoghurt

1 Simply mix all the ingredients together in a large bowl, and then transfer to a storage container. For one serving, remove 2-3 heaped tablespoons (about 60g/2 oz) of muesli from the container and soak in water, apple juice, milk or a dairy-free alternative, preferably overnight. If you can't remember to soak it the night before, even soaking it for a few minutes makes it much more digestible. Add other ingredients as your blood sugar level and your taste dictate.

Note: I have deliberately not included dried fruit in this, as it's better to use fresh fruit when possible, but you could add a few raisins or chopped dried apricots or figs if your blood sugar is normal. Fresh berries, chopped apple or pear, plums or cherries are all good low GI fruit to add. As for oats and oat bran, they are good for the health of the arteries. The soluble fibre they contain helps to reduce harmful levels of cholesterol in the blood. Jumbo oats are particularly valuable for people with diabetes as they have been minimally processed and therefore take longer to digest than quick-cooking porridge oats. Wholegrains, such as oats, should always be soaked (or cooked) before eating, as this breaks down the enzyme inhibitors that they contain.

The original muesli was invented in 1900 by Swiss doctor Maximilian Bircher-Benner for his patients, and consisted of rolled oats soaked in water, lemon juice, cream or yoghurt and a grated apple, perhaps topped with chopped or ground hazelnuts or almonds. Muesli has come a long way since those days, and not always in the right direction. This is my own diabetes-friendly version. For celiacs, oats certified as gluten-free can be obtained from Tilquhillie Fine Foods (see Useful Addresses).

Per Serving:
Calories (kcal) 250.2
Protein (g) 10.8
Carbohydrates (g) 28.6
Total Sugars (g) 3.1
Dietary Fibre (g) 6.5
Total Fat (g) 13.0
Saturated Fat (g) 1.5

42% carbohydrate, GL: Ⓜ

This is a sophisticated variation on Scotland's national breakfast dish. This porridge is eaten cold, topped with a raspberry purée – ideal for warm summer mornings. Other berries can be substituted for the raspberries – blueberries and strawberries work well.

fresh raspberry porridge

Serves 4 **Time taken:** 15 minutes

225g/8 oz (1²/₃ cups) Fresh or frozen and thawed raspberries
1 Orange, juice only
45g/1¹/₂ oz (¹/₂ cup) Jumbo oats
450ml/ 16 fl oz (2 cups) Milk or dairy-free alternative
4 tbsp Strained Greek yoghurt or soya yoghurt
Garnish A few whole raspberries

1 Start the night before you mean to serve the porridge. Put the raspberries and orange juice in a blender and blend to a purée. If you prefer the purée without seeds, you can sieve it to make it even smoother. Chill overnight. Put the oats into a thick bottomed pan with the milk and bring to the boil, stirring. Reduce the heat and simmer for 3-5 minutes, stirring frequently, until the porridge is smooth. Remove from the heat, leave to cool, and then chill overnight.

2 In the morning, stir the yoghurt into the chilled porridge, then divide between four glass serving bowls. Top with the raspberry purée and garnish with a few whole raspberries.

Note: Raspberries contain a little iron together with a lot of vitamin C, which helps your body absorb the iron. Like all berries, they are relatively low GI, thus causing only a slow increase in blood glucose.

Per Serving:
Calories (kcal) 147.7
Protein (g) 7.4
Carbohydrates (g) 24.0
Total Sugars (g) 3.5
Dietary Fibre (g) 4.8
Fat (g) 3.5
Saturated Fat (g) 1.9

61% carbohydrate, GL: M

scottish groats with cinnamon and raisins

Serves 2 **Time taken:** 1^1/$_2$ hours plus soaking

6 tbsp Oat groats
600ml/1 pt (2^1/$_2$ cups) Water
1 tsp Cinnamon
2 tbsp Raisins
Milk or dairy-free alternative, to serve

1 Wash the oat groats, then soak for several hours in cold water. I usually do this during the day. When you are ready to cook the groats, transfer to a saucepan together with the soaking water, and bring to the boil. Lower the heat to a simmer, and cook for 1-1^1/$_2$ hours, or until cooked to your liking, adding more water as necessary. This can be done the night before, then left to cool and reheated at breakfast time.

2 Alternatively, the groats can be successfully cooked overnight in the low oven of an Aga or on the low setting of an electric slow cooker.

3 Before serving the groats, stir in the cinnamon and raisins.
Serve with milk of your choice.

Note: Cinnamon is one of the most therapeutic spices for diabetics. It has been shown in studies to reduce blood glucose levels in people with Type 2 diabetes. You need ^{1}/$_2$ tsp per day, every day, to get this blood-sugar lowering effect. There are several other recipes in this book featuring cinnamon.

Oat groats look a little like brown rice grains. They are in fact whole oats that haven't been crushed and rolled. They have to be soaked overnight and cooked for a long time, but they are well worth the trouble. Apparently the late Queen Mother ate oat groats for breakfast every morning, which may have explained her longevity.

Per Serving:
Calories (kcal) 149.0
Protein (g) 4.3
Carbohydrates (g) 30.3
Total Sugars (g) 7.2
Dietary Fibre (g) 1.2
Fat (g) 1.9
Saturated Fat (g) 0.0

42% carbohydrate, GL: ⬤ Ⓜ ⬤

The standard Spanish tortilla is always made with potatoes and often served in little squares at tapas bars, or cut into wedges for a light meal. Using green vegetables in place of the potatoes makes it lighter and more suitable for breakfast. Spanish cooks flip their tortillas after browning the underside, but being a coward I usually finish mine off under the grill.

Per Serving:
Calories (kcal) 200.3
Protein (g) 10.2
Carbohydrates (g) 9.1
Total Sugars (g) 3.4
Dietary Fibre (g) 2.4
Fat (g) 13.7
Saturated Fat (g) 3.1

tortilla paisana

Serves 4 **Time taken:** 30 minutes

6 Fresh free-range eggs
Sea salt and freshly ground black pepper
2 tbsp Extra virgin olive oil
1 large Mild onion, peeled and chopped
100g/3¹/₂ oz (1 cup) Cooked green beans
100g/3¹/₂ oz (1 cup) Cooked peas (or thawed frozen peas)
1 Courgette, sliced

1 Beat the eggs with a little seasoning. Heat the olive oil in a large frying pan, preferably one that is 23cm/9" in diameter for a 6-egg tortilla. Add the chopped onion and cook over gentle heat until the onion is soft. Add the rest of the vegetables, and then the beaten eggs. Cook over gentle heat until the bottom is set. Don't try to rush this part – it may take up to 15 minutes or so. Meanwhile, heat the grill. When the tortilla is beginning to firm up, take the pan off the heat and slide it under the grill to set and cook the top side. When the tortilla is cooked through, slide out onto a plate and cut into wedges and serve warm. Any leftovers can be eaten at room temperature with salad for a light meal.

Variations: you can use any green vegetables for this, such as steamed asparagus tips, broccoli spears or spinach.

61% carbohydrate, GL: **M**

pipérade

Serves 4 **Time taken:** 20 minutes

2 **Sweet peppers, red, green or orange**
2 tbsp **Extra virgin olive oil**
4 **Cloves garlic (optional)**
1 small **Onion, finely chopped**
2 large **Tomatoes, peeled, seeded and chopped**
8 **Free-range eggs, beaten**
Sea salt and freshly ground black pepper

1 Roast the peppers under the grill until charred, then pop them into a paper bag
or wrap them in a cloth for a few minutes – this makes them easier to peel.
Peel off the outer skin. Discard the seeds and cut into strips. Heat the oil in a large
frying pan and sauté the chopped garlic, if using, and onion. Add the peeled and
chopped tomatoes with the strips of pepper and fry for about 15 minutes, until some of
the liquid has evaporated. Turn into a bowl and set aside (this can be done the previous
evening).

2 Heat a little oil in the pan and pour in the eggs. Stir over a very gentle heat
until barely set, as for scrambled eggs. Reheat the pepper and tomato mixture
if necessary, and stir into the eggs. Season to taste and serve immediately.
The success of this dish depends on not overcooking the eggs, or it becomes watery
and grainy. When perfectly made it is creamy and delectable.

**Note: Peppers are one of the best sources of vitamin C, but this vitamin is easily
damaged by light, air and storage, so buy your vegetables as fresh as possible,
consume them quickly and don't cut them up too soon before eating.**

This egg dish originated
in the Basque country,
where it is known as
Piperrada, but it has been
incorporated into French
cuisine over the years.
4 cloves of garlic might
be too much for breakfast,
so feel free to use less,
or leave it out entirely.

Per Serving:
Calories (kcal) 280.8
Protein (g) 10.1
Carbohydrates (g) 11.3
Total Sugars (g) 5.9
Dietary Fibre (g) 2.4
Fat (g) 21.9
Saturated Fat (g) 4.2

16% carbohydrate, GL: Ⓛ ● ●

eggs with yoghurt

This is a Bulgarian dish usually eaten as a main meal. As long as you have the time to bake it, it's very quick to put together, admirably high in protein and low in carbohydrate, so it's ideal for when your blood sugar is high in the morning yet you know you need to eat breakfast.

Serves 2 **Time taken:** 15 minutes

Butter, for greasing
300ml/^{1}/$_2$ pt (1^1/$_4$ cups) Natural live yoghurt (see page 140)
4 Free-range eggs
110g/4 oz Labneh (see page 141)
60g/2 oz (^{3}/$_4$ cup) Fresh wholemeal, rye or gluten-free breadcrumbs
Sea salt and freshly ground black pepper
Fresh berries, to serve

1 Preheat the oven to 180°C/350°F/gas 4. Butter a baking dish.

2 Beat together all the other ingredients. This can be done in the liquidizer or by hand. Pour the mixture into the prepared baking dish, and bake in the preheated oven until firm and golden. Serve with fresh berries – this is not traditional but it balances the dish well.

Note: This dish is high in dairy products, but if you choose your dairy products wisely, that should not be a problem. Make your home-made yoghurt with organic milk, which recent research has shown to be higher in Omega 3 fatty acids than regular milk. Many people can tolerate yoghurt and labneh where they can't tolerate milk, because the bacteria in these fermented foods have pre-digested the lactose (milk sugar) present in milk, thus making it more digestible.

Per Serving:
Calories (kcal) 338.7
Protein (g) 25.0
Carbohydrates (g) 29.9
Total Sugars (g) 2.0
Dietary Fibre (g) 2.0
Fat (g) 13.7
Saturated Fat (g) 5.2

35% carbohydrate, GL: M

iranian herb kuku

Serves 4 **Time taken:** 15 minutes

15g/¹/₂ oz (1 tbsp) Organic unsalted butter
6 Free-range eggs, beaten
1 large bunch Fresh flat-leaf parsley, washed and chopped
1 large bunch Fresh coriander, washed and chopped
1 large bunch Fresh chives, washed and chopped
Sea salt and freshly ground black pepper
1 tbsp Dried currants
2 tbsp Walnuts, coarsely chopped

1 Heat the butter in a large, heavy frying pan. Stir the herbs into the beaten eggs, season to taste and stir in the currants and walnuts. Pour into the frying pan and cook over a gentle heat until set. Slide onto a large plate and return to the pan bottom side up to cook the other side. If you feel unconfident about doing this, the top can be browned under a grill instead.

Note: In these quantities, fresh herbs deliver a nutritional kick. Usually used as a garnish, parsley is very high in vitamin C (20g provides the recommended daily amount for an adult), coriander is rich in selenium, and chives, being a member of the onion family, contain allicin which is an immune-booster.

According to Claudia Roden, this is the ancestor of the Spanish tortilla and the Italian frittata. The success of this dish relies on the freshness and quantity of the herbs used, so don't try it with herbs from supermarket plastic packs.

Per Serving:
Calories (kcal) 162.83
Protein (g) 9.86
Carbohydrates (g) 4.3
Total Sugars (g) 2.0
Dietary Fibre (g) 1.31
Fat (g) 11.96
Saturated Fat (g) 4.06

10% carbohydrate, GL: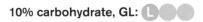

You often see this dish on 'Tex-Mex' menus in the United States. It's quick to make if you already have the sauce in the fridge, where it will keep for up to 3 days.

huevos rancheros

Serves 6 **Time taken:** 30 minutes

1 recipe Mexican Salsa Picante (see page 145)
6 Fresh free-range eggs
6 Corn tortillas

1 Preheat the oven to 180°C/350°F/gas 4. Pour the salsa into a 30cm x 20cm/12" x 8" baking dish.

2 Make 6 indentations in the sauce, and break an egg into each. Bake in the preheated oven until the eggs are set – about 15 minutes. Meanwhile, wrap the tortillas in foil and heat in the oven alongside the egg dish. Serve the eggs immediately, accompanied by hot tortillas.

Note: Corn tortillas are gluten-free, so they are a useful starchy food for celiacs. In Mexico, corn tortillas are the most widely consumed staple food. The corn dough used for tortilla preparation, masa harina, is traditionally prepared by boiling corn in a lime solution, and letting it stand overnight. In this country you can buy corn tortillas ready made in most supermarkets. To heat, either wrap in foil and heat for 10 minutes in a hot oven, or fry briefly in hot oil.

Per Serving:
Calories (kcal) 177.7
Protein (g) 7.5
Carbohydrates (g) 19.3
Total Sugars (g) 2.7
Dietary Fibre (g) 1.8
Fat (g) 7.8
Saturated Fat (g) 1.7

43% carbohydrate, GL: M

cornmeal turkish-style (kacamak)

Serves 3 **Time taken:** 15 minutes

110g/4 oz ($^1/_2$ cup) **Yellow cornmeal or polenta**
450ml/16 fl oz (2 cups) **Water**
1 tbsp **Extra virgin olive oil**
$^1/_2$ tsp **Sea salt**
60g/2 oz (4 tbsp) **Organic unsalted butter**
60g/2 oz (4 tbsp) **Canned tomatoes, chopped**
Feta cheese, crumbled

1 Bring the water, olive oil and salt to a rolling boil in a heavy based saucepan. Slowly pour in the cornmeal, stirring constantly. Continue to stir and cook over low heat for 10-12 minutes making sure there are no lumps. The mixture should thicken and start to leave the sides of the pot when it is cooked. Meanwhile, melt the butter in a small pan and heat the chopped tomato gently in it. When ready to serve, place the kacamak on a warmed plate and pour the tomatoes over it. Sprinkle on some crumbled feta cheese and serve hot.

Note: Corn is a significant source of dietary fibre and supplies many minerals such as potassium and magnesium as well as B vitamins. It is also, of course, a gluten-free grain, so ideal for celiacs.

This is an easy and appetizing cornmeal dish served in Turkey and the Balkans for breakfast. It is traditionally stirred and mashed with a kacamas, a specially designed large flat wooden spoon a little like a potato masher.

Per Serving:
Calories (kcal) 325.6
Protein (g) 4.1
Carbohydrates (g) 29.2
Total Sugars (g) 0.5
Dietary Fibre (g) 3.5
Fat (g) 22.2
Saturated Fat (g) 12.6

42% carbohydrate, GL: ● Ⓜ ●

buckwheat blinis with creamed kippers

Blinis are little yeasted buckwheat pancakes, traditionally eaten in Russia with sour cream and caviar. It's quite easy to make them using the little sachets of instant yeast so readily available nowadays, but you do need to factor in half an hour resting time, so this is a recipe for weekends and holidays.

Per Serving:
Calories (kcal) 406.9
Protein (g) 21.1
Carbohydrates (g) 30.6
Total Sugars (g) 1.7
Dietary Fibre (g) 5.4
Fat (g) 21.7
Saturated Fat (g) 8.7

Makes 16 **Time taken:** 30 minutes

For the topping: 170g/6 oz Kipper fillets, boned, cooked and flaked
4 tbsp Greek yoghurt or plain soya yoghurt
1 level tbsp Chopped chives
$1/2$ tsp Finely grated lemon rind
Freshly ground black pepper
For the blinis: 45g/$1^1/2$ oz (3 tbsp) Organic unsalted butter
175ml/6 fl oz ($3/4$ cup) Milk or dairy-free alternative
100g/$3^1/2$ oz ($2/3$ cup) Buckwheat flour
75g/$2^1/2$ oz ($1/3$ cup) Rice flour
$2^1/2$ tsp Fast-acting dried yeast (1 sachet)
2 Free-range eggs, separated
Extra virgin olive oil or clarified butter for frying

1 For the blinis, melt the butter in a small pan, then stir in the milk. Set aside.
Mix together the buckwheat flour, rice flour and yeast in a large bowl and make a well in the centre. Put the egg yolks and milk and butter mixture into the well. Stir to incorporate the flour into a smooth batter. Cover the bowl and set aside for half an hour while you make the topping.

2 For the topping, mix the cooked flaked kipper with the Greek yoghurt or soya yoghurt, chopped chives and lemon rind. Season with freshly ground black pepper. Set aside.

3 Beat the egg whites until stiff, then fold them into the batter using a metal spoon. Heat a little oil or clarified butter in a large frying pan over medium heat. Carefully pour the batter into the pan in spoonfuls, to make small pancakes about 6cm in diameter, about 3-4 at a time, depending on the size of the pan. When their undersides are brown, turn the blinis over with a palette knife to cook the other side. Remove from the pan and keep warm, covered with a cloth, while you cook the remainder of the batter.

4 To serve, top each blini with a dollop of the kipper mixture and serve 4 per person.

Note: Buckwheat is beneficial for people with diabetes for a number of reasons. It has a low GI (although buckwheat flour is higher than whole buckwheat grains), and it contains chiro-inositol which appears to prompt cells to become more insulin-sensitive. It also contains rutin which aids circulation. The inclusion of both kippers and dairy products mean that this dish is especially high in calcium (107mg per serving).

30% carbohydrate, GL:

korean mung bean pancakes

Serves 4 Time taken: 30 minutes

200g/7 oz (1 cup) Dried mung beans, soaked overnight
2 Garlic cloves
1 Free-range egg, beaten
Handful of mung bean sprouts
60g/2 oz (1/2 cup) Chinese cabbage or bok choy, coarsely chopped
4 Spring onions, finely chopped
Freshly ground black pepper
1 tbsp Groundnut oil, for frying
To serve: Tamari (Japanese soy sauce)

1 Grind the beans and garlic cloves with about 225ml/8 fl oz/1 cup water in a blender until smooth. Add the beaten egg, a little at a time, to get a fairly thick batter.

2 Just before you want to make the pancakes, mix in the bean sprouts, Chinese cabbage or bok choy, spring onions and pepper (you don't need salt as the pancakes will be dipped in soy sauce, which is salty enough). Heat a griddle or thick-bottomed frying pan, wipe with a piece of kitchen paper dipped in groundnut oil, and drop spoonfuls of the batter into the pan. Cook until small bubbles appear on the surface, then flip and cook the other side. Keep warm, covered with a tea towel, while you cook the rest of the batter. Serve with tamari sauce for dipping.

Note: Mung beans are exceptionally low GI, so these make a very diabetic-friendly breakfast. Soy beans, canned chickpeas, yellow split peas or red lentils could be substituted for the mung beans.

These pancakes, known as *Bindae Duk*, are eaten for breakfast in Korea. They often contain shredded pork or beef and are dipped in soy sauce at the table.
This is a lighter vegetarian version.

Per Serving:
Calories (kcal) 230.5
Protein (g) 14.4
Carbohydrates (g) 31.5
Total Sugars (g) 0.3
Dietary Fibre (g) 9.9
Fat (g) 5.3
Saturated Fat (g) 0.9

55% carbohydrate, GL: **M**

egg and herring open sandwiches

Serves 4 **Time taken:** 15 minutes

4 slices Black rye bread (pumpernickel)
Organic unsalted butter
4 Free-range eggs
2 tbsp Milk or dairy-free alternative
Sea salt and freshly ground black pepper
1 tbsp Sour cream or soya yoghurt
4 Pickled herring fillets, flat or rolled
A few thin onion rings
4 Small wedges of lemon
Sprigs of dill or fennel

1 Spread each slice of black rye bread with butter. Beat the eggs with the milk and seasoning. Heat 15g/^{1}/$_2$ oz/1 tbsp butter in a pan, add the egg mixture and cook over a gentle heat, stirring continuously until the eggs are just set but still creamy. Remove from the heat and stir in the sour cream or soya yoghurt. Allow to cool. Spoon the eggs onto the buttered bread. Top with a herring fillet, a couple of small onion rings, a lemon wedge and a sprig of dill or fennel.

Note: It is a shame that we eat so few herrings these days. They are the only oily fish with a favourable EPA/DHA ratio (this is thought to be especially good for the heart), and the best source of vitamin D. There is more and more evidence emerging that points to vitamin D deficiency as having a critical role in the development of diabetes and other chronic diseases, as well as being endemic in the older population.

These are typical Danish fare, known as Smørrebrød (literally, 'butter on bread').
There are hundreds of toppings for open sandwiches, but this combination of scrambled eggs and pickled herring is often eaten for breakfast. It is a very well balanced meal, high in protein, especially useful if you've woken up with high blood sugar but need to eat something before heading out.

Per Serving:
Calories (kcal) 241.9
Protein (g) 12.7
Carbohydrates (g) 15.6
Total Sugars (g) 1.1
Dietary Fibre (g) 1.7
Fat (g) 14.1
Saturated Fat (g) 4.2

26% carbohydrate, GL: Ⓛ ○ ○

kao tom (thai breakfast soup)

Serves 4 **Time taken:** 15 minutes

1 litre/1³/₄ pts (4 cups) Chicken stock, preferably home made
225g/¹/₂ lb (1 cup) Cooked chicken, shredded
200g/7 oz (1 cup) Cooked brown rice
4 Organic free-range eggs
2 tbsp Cider vinegar
Nam Pla (Thai fish sauce) to taste
Optional garnishes: Chopped chillies, grated fresh ginger, chopped spring onion,
    chopped coriander leaves

1 In a medium saucepan, bring chicken stock to a rolling boil. Add the shredded
chicken and cooked rice. Reduce the heat to low, cover and simmer for at least five
minutes, stirring occasionally, until the chicken is thoroughly reheated.

2 While the soup is simmering, poach the eggs: fill a deep saucepan with water, add a
couple of tablespoons of vinegar and bring to the boil. Reduce the heat so that the
water is just simmering, break the first egg into a cup, stir the simmering water
vigorously with a wooden spoon, then slip the egg into the water to poach for about 4
minutes. Lift out with a slotted spoon and drain on paper towels. Keep warm. Repeat
with the other eggs.

3 To serve, reheat the soup to boiling and add Nam Pla to taste. Put a poached egg into
each of 4 bowls, and ladle the hot soup on top of the eggs. Garnish with any or all of
the following, according to your taste: chopped chilli, grated ginger, chopped spring
onion, chopped coriander leaves.

**Note: Thai cooks break a raw egg into each bowl and let the hot soup cook the
egg. For reasons of food safety I prefer to poach the eggs first.**

Kao Tom is the traditional breakfast in Thailand, but it may also accompany other meals too. It can be cooked plain, or with seafood, pork or chicken, as here. It is almost always made from rice cooked the previous day, although the rice can be cooked slowly in the broth – this will make a thicker soup, almost like a porridge. As elsewhere, I have substituted brown rice for the usual white rice to lighten the glycaemic load.

Per Serving:
Calories (kcal) 128.9
Protein (g) 13.6
Carbohydrates (g) 15
Total Sugars (g) 1.2
Dietary Fibre (g) 1.9
Fat (g) 1.5
Saturated Fat (g) 0.1

47% carbohydrate, GL: **M**

american carrot and courgette muffins

Makes 12 muffins **Time taken:** 45 minutes

The Americans have perfected this quickly baked treat. Sadly, however, most muffins are far too high in refined flour and sugar to be considered diabetic-friendly. These muffins, on the other hand, are made with wholemeal flour and rely on concentrated apple juice and spices for sweetness and on vegetables for taste and added fibre.

Unsalted butter for greasing
285g/10 oz (2 cups) Wholemeal flour
2 tsp Baking powder
1 tsp Ground cinnamon
1/2 tsp Ground nutmeg
1/2 tsp Ground ginger
1/4 tsp Sea salt
225ml/6 fl oz (3/4 cup) Milk or dairy-free alternative
75ml/21/2 fl oz (1/3 cup) Concentrated apple juice
75ml/21/2 fl oz (1 cup) Extra virgin olive oil
2 Free-range eggs
1 tsp Vanilla extract
1 large Courgette, grated
2 medium Carrots, finely grated

1 Preheat the oven to 190°C/375°F/gas 5.

2 Butter a 12-cup muffin tin, or use a non-stick muffin tin. In a large mixing bowl, combine the flour, baking powder, spices and salt. In a small bowl, whisk together the milk, apple juice, oil, eggs, and vanilla.

3 Stir the milk mixture into the dry ingredients just until the flour is moistened. The batter will be lumpy, but successful muffins depend on a very light hand. Squeeze the grated vegetables with your hands to extract any liquid, and then fold them into the batter. Divide the batter between the muffin cups.

4 Bake for 25 to 30 minutes, or until the centres spring back when lightly touched with a finger. Cool in the pan on a rack for 5 minutes before turning out.

5 Serve with fromage frais, if liked.

Note: These muffins contain cinnamon, one of the 'superfoods' for diabetics as it can help to lower blood sugar.

Per Serving:
Calories (kcal) 179.9
Protein (g) 5.4
Carbohydrates (g) 21.8
Total Sugars (g) 3.5
Dietary Fibre (g) 3.3
Fat (g) 7.9
Saturated Fat (g) 1.5

48% carbohydrate, GL:

english country garden juice

Serves 2 **Time taken:** 5 minutes

2 medium Organic carrots, scrubbed but not peeled
1 Uncooked beetroot, peeled
1/2 Cucumber
1 Handful of spinach
2 Cloves of garlic
2 Parsley sprigs
1/2 Lemon, peeled

1 Cut all the vegetables so that they fit into the juicer. Juice all the ingredients and drink immediately.

Variation: **try replacing the garlic with a 2.5cm/1" piece of peeled ginger root.**

Note: **Beetroot is a rich source of folate, which can help to reduce the risk of heart disease. Adequate intakes of folate appear to decrease levels of homocysteine, a toxic bi-product of protein metabolism which, when raised, is a significant cardiovascular disease risk factor.**

Fruit juice for breakfast is not a good idea for anyone with diabetes, as it's a very concentrated sugar. However, vegetable juice is another matter, delivering quality nutrition in a glass. This juice includes vegetables that might be found in a typical kitchen garden.

Per Serving:
Calories (kcal) 62.9
Protein (g) 2.8
Carbohydrates (g) 14.4
Total Sugars (g) 1.1
Dietary Fibre (g) 1.2
Fat (g) 0.2
Saturated Fat (g) 0.0

81% carbohydrate, GL: ● Ⓜ ●

Mango lassi is the traditional Indian breakfast drink. The relatively high GI of the mango is tempered by the protein and fat in the yoghurt. However, it still scores a fairly high glycaemic load, so proceed carefully, perhaps having a protein food afterwards, such as a handful of nuts, a piece of smoked fish or a poached egg.

mango lassi

Serves 2 **Time taken:** 5 minutes

255g/ 9 oz (1/2 pound) **Ripe mango**
150ml /5 fl oz (2/3 cup) **Milk or dairy-free alternative**
150ml /5 fl oz (2/3 cup) **Natural live yoghurt (see page 140) or soya yoghurt**
1/4 tsp **Ground cardamom (optional)**

1 Peel the mango and put the pulp into the blender. Blend until smooth then push through a sieve to get rid of any fibres. Put back into the blender with the milk, yoghurt and cardamom if using, and blend together.

Note: Mangoes are a good source of potassium, which is a key mineral for people suffering from high blood pressure. A whole mango supplies one third of an adult's daily potassium requirement.

Per Serving:
Calories (kcal) 167.4
Protein (g) 7.8
Carbohydrates (g) 29.5
Total Sugars (g) 16.8
Dietary Fibre (g) 1.0
Fat (g) 3.1
Saturated Fat (g) 1.8

67% carbohydrate, GL: M

papaya and coconut smoothie

Serves 2 **Time taken:** 5 minutes

1 Ripe papaya, peeled, seeded and cut into chunks
2 Oranges, juiced
$1/2$ Banana, cut into chunks
90g/3 oz Silken tofu
60ml /2 fl oz (4 tbsp) Coconut milk
1 tsp Grated root ginger

1 Put the papaya, orange juice, banana, tofu, coconut milk and root ginger into the blender. Blend until smooth and serve immediately. This is also very refreshing on a hot day if you freeze the papaya chunks and banana first.

Note: Papayas are particularly rich in vitamin C and are also a useful source of antioxidants and fibre. They also contain an enzyme called papain which breaks down protein. In Chinese medicine, papayas have traditionally been given to those who find it difficult to digest protein-rich foods.

I love the tropical taste of this smoothie, which reminds me of when I lived in the Caribbean. The combination of papaya, orange juice and banana delivers quite a high glycaemic load, which is why I've added some tofu. It would be wise to eat a protein food alongside this too, such as poached or scrambled eggs without the toast, or a piece of fish.

Per Serving:
Calories (kcal) 205.4
Protein (g) 4.6
Carbohydrates (g) 32.9
Total Sugars (g) 20.4
Dietary Fibre (g) 4.1
Fat (g) 7.7
Saturated Fat (g) 5.6

60% carbohydrate, GL: M

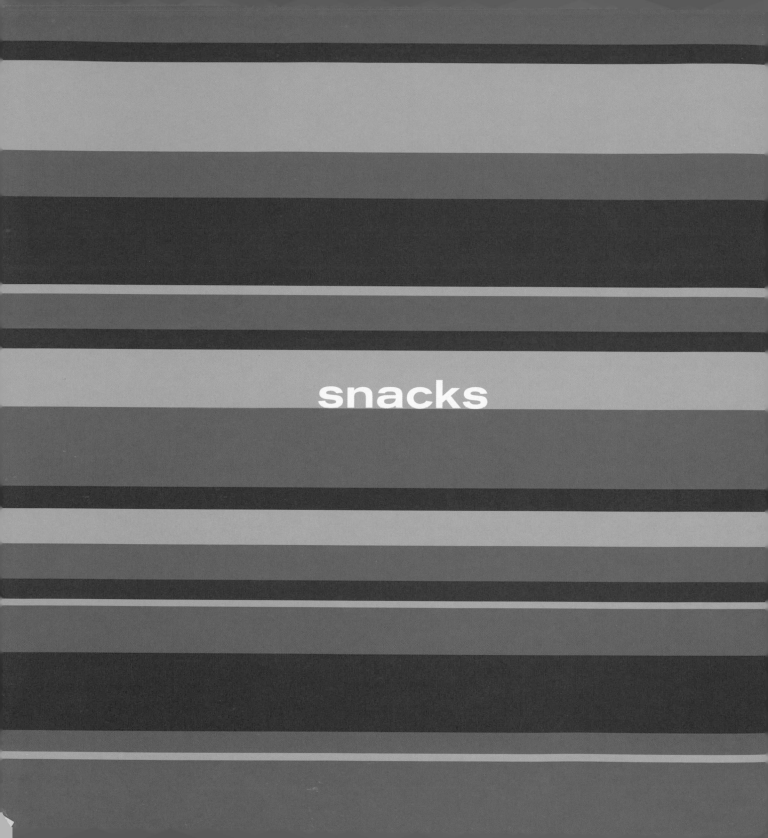

snacks

Snacks are very important for diabetics as a means of keeping the blood sugar even between meals. Many culinary traditions, such as the tapas of Spain and the mezze of the Middle East, answer this need perfectly. To qualify for inclusion in this chapter, a recipe had to be either very quick to make or able to be made in advance and eaten straight from the fridge with the minimum of last-minute preparation. Many of these are 'go-anywhere' snacks – foods that you can stash in your bag and take with you to munch on during the day. The other important criterion is that a snack should have a good balance of protein and carbohydrate. That's where dips and spreads come in handy, as it is easy to incorporate a protein food such as fish, cheese or beans into a dip or spread, and eat it with a carbohydrate food such as crackers or vegetable sticks.

Ideal snacks that need no cooking are:

- A piece of low GI fruit and a handful of nuts
- Hummus with crudités
- Toast or crackers with nut butter
- Mashed beans or cold dahl (see page 95) with raw vegetables
- Natural yoghurt with berries and a sprinkling of sunflower seeds
- Pumpkin seeds lightly roasted or dry fried and sprinkled with tamari sauce

Leftovers make good snacks too. Leftovers of the following recipes are easily portable and can be eaten as cold snacks:

- Tortilla paisana (page 32)
- Greek courgette cakes (page 72)
- Buckwheat blinis (page 38)
- American carrot and courgette muffins (page 42)
- Lentil rolls (page 138)
- Tofu and coriander cakes (page 75)

This is a typical Spanish tapa. The almonds can be made in quantity and stored in an airtight tin or jar for instant snacking.

spanish-style toasted almonds

Serves 16 **Time taken:** 20 minutes

450g/1lb Almonds in their skins
1 tbsp Extra virgin olive oil
Sea salt
Paprika

1 Preheat the oven to 200°C/400°F/gas 6.

2 Blanch the almonds very briefly in boiling water, drain and slip off the skins while still warm. Dry well on kitchen paper. Spread the almonds on a baking tray. Drizzle with olive oil, sprinkle with sea salt and a little paprika and toast in the oven, stirring frequently, just until slightly coloured.

Variation: the almonds can be toasted in a little olive oil in a frying pan.

Note: Almonds are high in vitamin E and are one of the richest non-animal sources of calcium. They have been shown to reduce total cholesterol, too. One study showed that after including almonds in the diet for three weeks, low-density lipoprotein (LDL) had decreased by 10%.

Per Serving:
Calories (kcal) 182
Protein (g) 6
Carbohydrates (g) 5.3
Total Sugars (g) 1.1
Dietary Fibre (g) 3.8
Fat (g) 15.2
Saturated Fat (g) 0.1

11% carbohydrate, GL: L ● ●

spicy chickpeas

Serves 16 **Time taken:** 50 minutes plus overnight soaking

450g/ 1lb (2 cups) Dried chickpeas
1/2 tsp Sea salt
1/2 tsp Ground cumin
1/2 tsp Ground coriander
1/2 tsp Cayenne pepper, or to taste

1 Soak the chickpeas overnight in plenty of cold water. The next day, drain thoroughly, and cook until not quite tender. Depending on the age of the chickpeas, this could take 1 1/2-2 hours. Drain and blot dry.

2 Spread the chickpeas in a single layer on a baking tray or trays. Bake in the preheated oven until golden-brown and crisp (about 30 minutes).

3 Toss with the salt and spices while still hot, tasting as you go to make sure you don't over-season. Store in an airtight tin or in the freezer.

Variation: these are also delicious sprinkled with Dukkah (see page 150).

Note: Chickpeas have a low GI – the average of four different studies was 28. Like other pulses, they are digested slowly and are therefore very valuable to people with diabetes. Over the long term they may help to improve blood glucose control.

These baked chickpeas are eaten in many different countries as a snack. I make them in large quantities and keep them in the freezer, just bringing out a handful at a time as needed. Don't be tempted to use canned chickpeas for this as they are too soft. You want them not quite cooked through so that they still have a little 'bite'.

Per Serving:
Calories (kcal) 95.9
Protein (g) 5.2
Carbohydrates (g) 16
Total Sugars (g) 2.8
Dietary Fibre (g) 4.5
Fat (g) 1.5
Saturated Fat (g) 0.2

65% carbohydrate, GL: M

The guacamole I have eaten in Mexico is coarsely chopped and fiery with chilli – a far cry from the bland smooth paste sold in British supermarkets. It takes moments to make your own and it's so much tastier.

guacamole

Serves 6 **Time taken:** 15 minutes

2 large Ripe avocados
1 Lime, juice only
1 large Ripe tomato, peeled, deseeded and diced
$1/2$ small Onion, peeled and finely chopped
1 Fresh green chilli, deseeded and finely chopped
1 tbsp Chopped fresh coriander
Sea salt

1 Halve the avocados and remove the stones. Mash the flesh with a fork and immediately stir in the lime juice to stop the avocado turning brown. Add the remaining ingredients and mix well. Season and serve immediately. If you are going to have to keep it for a bit, burying one of the avocado stones in the mixture and covering it seems to arrest discolouration.

Note: Avocados are rich in essential fatty acids, vitamin B6 and vitamin E, which is particularly valuable as a fat-soluble antioxidant which protects cholesterol from free radical damage. While many foods contain vitamin E, much of it is destroyed by cooking. Avocados have the advantage of requiring no processing.

Per Serving:
Calories (kcal) 150.0
Protein (g) 2.2
Carbohydrates (g) 11.0
Total Sugars (g) 2.4
Dietary Fibre (g) 6.3
Fat (g) 12.4
Saturated Fat (g) 1.8

27% carbohydrate, GL: Ⓛ ●●

lebanese aubergine dip

Serves 6-8 **Time taken:** 20 minutes

2 large Aubergines
2 Garlic cloves, peeled and finely chopped
Sea salt
1 tsp Ground cumin
Freshly ground black pepper
1 small Lemon, juice only
6 tbsp Extra virgin olive oil
2 tbsp Natural live yoghurt (see page 140)
1 tbsp Tahini

Preheat the grill and grill the aubergines, turning as the skin chars and the whole vegetables start to sag. Remove from the grill and set aside until cool enough to handle.

Meanwhile, crush the garlic with a little salt, using the back of a knife. Transfer to the food processor. Cut open the aubergines and scrape out the flesh into the food processor. Add the cumin, black pepper, half the lemon juice and half the olive oil. Process until smooth. Taste and adjust the flavour using olive oil, salt and lemon juice to taste. Add the yoghurt and tahini and process briefly. Serve as a dip with grilled or raw vegetables. It's also good as a sauce with grilled lamb.

Note: Aubergines are an excellent source of dietary fibre, with 2.5g of fibre per 100g. They are also a very good source of B vitamins and potassium.

This luscious dip is often served in Lebanese restaurants, where it is known as Moutabal.
It's less oily than hummus, and has a lovely smoky flavour, which comes from grilling or roasting the aubergines until they are scorched and the flesh is tender.

Per Serving:
Calories (kcal) 193.8
Protein (g) 2.8
Carbohydrates (g) 12.7
Total Sugars (g) 0.2
Dietary Fibre (g) 0.4
Fat (g) 15.8
Saturated Fat (g) 2.3

25% carbohydrate, GL: Ⓛ ●●

macedonian red pepper dip (htipti)

The translation of Htipiti is "that which is beaten". The longer it is beaten, the more tart this dip will be. Note, however, if you are restricting sodium, that feta cheese is salty. You could replace it with a less salty cheese such as ricotta, but the taste will not be the same.

Serves 10 **Time taken:** 15 minutes

3 Red peppers
1 Fresh red chilli, deseeded and roughly chopped
340g/12 oz Feta cheese, crumbled
1 Garlic clove, peeled and roughly chopped
4-6 tbsp Extra virgin olive oil
To serve: Paprika

1 First, grill the red peppers under a hot grill, turning once or twice, until the skin is scorched and blackened. Leave until cool enough to handle, then skin and deseed the peppers, and chop roughly.

2 Place all the ingredients in a food processor or blender. Blend until very smooth, adding enough olive oil to give a thick dipping consistency. Season to taste, then spoon into a serving bowl and serve sprinkled with paprika and accompanied by raw vegetables for dipping.

3 This dip, which can also be used as a sauce on meat, fish or vegetables, keeps for up to three days covered in the refrigerator.

Note: Red peppers are one of the most nutrient-dense foods available. They are a fantastic source of vitamin C, although much of this is lost in cooking. They are also a very good source of phytochemicals with exceptional antioxidant activity. Studies have shown that they have a protective effect against cataracts as well as preventing blood clot formation.

Per Serving:
Calories (kcal) 157.9
Protein (g) 6.4
Carbohydrates (g) 3.4
Total Sugars (g) 1.3
Dietary Fibre (g) 1.7
Fat (g) 12.6
Saturated Fat (g) 4.6

9% carbohydrate, GL: L

tahini cream with almonds

Serves 6 **Time taken:** 15 minutes

1 Garlic clove, peeled
Sea salt
$2^1/_2$ - 3 Lemons, juice only
150ml/5 fl oz ($^2/_3$ cup) Tahini (sesame seed paste)
1 tsp Ground cumin
5 tbsp Ground almonds
5 whole Blanched almonds, for garnish
To serve: Crudités such as carrot sticks, celery sticks, slices of pepper

1 Crush the garlic with a little salt. Put into the blender with most of the lemon juice, the tahini, ground cumin, ground almonds and a little cold water. Process to a thick cream, adding more salt and/or lemon juice to taste and more cold water as necessary to achieve a good consistency and balance of flavours. Turn into a serving bowl, garnish with the whole blanched almonds and serve with crudités.

Note: This dip is very rich in minerals, particularly calcium and magnesium. Almonds are the richest vegetarian source of calcium, with sesame seeds a close second. Sesame seeds are a rich source of highly unsaturated oils, and are a perfect balance of potassium and sodium which helps the body to maintain normal blood pressure and a good fluid balance.

This is a subtle variation of the tahini cream salad served all over the Middle East as part of a mezze. It is usually eaten with pitta bread, but is also delicious eaten as a dip with raw vegetables. Tahini, if you've never tried it, is a sesame seed paste sold in health food shops, delicatessens and most supermarkets. There are light and dark versions, the former being made from hulled sesame seeds, whilst the latter is made from unhulled seeds.

Per Serving:
Calories (kcal) 193.1
Protein (g) 5.9
Carbohydrates (g) 9.0
Total Sugars (g) 0.9
Dietary Fibre (g) 2.1
Fat (g) 16.6

17% carbohydrate, GL: **L** ● ●

This spicy walnut dip is a little like hummus in texture. The original recipe called for pomegranate molasses, a thick, sweet-sour syrup which you can find in Middle Eastern shops, but which is expensive. If you can't find it, or are unwilling to buy a whole bottle when you only need a tablespoonful (as I am), you can use my makeshift substitution, which has the advantage of containing no added sugar.

Per Serving:
Calories (kcal) 240.1
Protein (g) 3.7
Carbohydrates (g) 15.8
Total Sugars (g) 9.7
Dietary Fibre (g) 2
Fat (g) 19.6
Saturated Fat (g) 2.3

walnut and red chilli dip (muhhamarra)

Serves 6 **Time taken:** 15 minutes

2 Pomegranates
1 Lemon, juice only
2 whole Dried red chillies, soaked in warm water for 30 minutes
90g/3 oz ($3/4$ cup) Chopped walnuts
2 Garlic cloves, peeled and finely chopped
45g/$1^1/2$ oz ($1/2$ cup) Fresh wholemeal, rye or gluten-free breadcrumbs
60ml/2 fl oz ($1/4$ cup) Extra virgin olive oil

1 First, prepare the pomegranates: Roll them on your work surface until they soften, then break them up under water to keep the juice from spurting. Give a good bang with the back of the knife to loosen the seeds of each section. To squeeze out the juice, wrap a handful of seeds in a cloth, then use your hands to squeeze into a bowl to obtain the rich, shiny liquid. Repeat with the remaining seeds. Put the pomegranate juice and lemon juice in a small pan and reduce by boiling until there is only a tablespoon left. Alternatively, use 3 tablespoons of bottled unsweetened pomegranate juice and 1 tablespoon of lemon juice and reduce to 1 tablespoon as above.

2 Drain the soaked chillies and discard the water. Combine all the ingredients including the red chillies and blend to a smooth paste. Serve with rye crispbread, oatcakes or raw vegetables.

Note: Walnuts, being a very good source of omega 3 fatty acids, reduce the risk of heart attacks in those who eat them regularly. Since diabetes increases your cardiovascular risk, it makes sense to eat walnuts regularly. If possible, buy them in the shell, as they oxidise easily on exposure to air.

25% carbohydrate, GL: ⬤⬤⬤

butter bean ta'amia

Serves 4 **Time taken:** 2 hours 15 minutes plus overnight soaking

110g/4 oz (²/₃ cup) Butter beans (lima beans)
1 large Onion, peeled and roughly chopped
2 Garlic cloves, peeled and chopped
1 tsp Coriander seeds
1 tsp Cumin seeds
1 tsp Fennel seeds
Small handful of parsley
¹/₂ tsp Baking powder
1 small Free-range egg, beaten
Sea salt and freshly ground black pepper
A little flour for flouring the hands
2 tbsp Extra virgin olive oil
To serve: Natural live yoghurt (see page 140)

1 Soak the dried beans overnight in cold water to cover. Drain, boil in fresh water for 10 minutes, then lower the heat, cover and simmer for 1¹/₂ - 2 hours, depending on the age of the beans. Drain. Alternatively, use one 400g/14 oz can of beans, drained and rinsed.

2 Preheat the oven to 200°C/400°F/gas 6. Grind the spices with a pestle and mortar or in an electric grinder.

3 Put the cooked beans, onion, garlic, ground spices, parsley and baking powder into a food processor or blender and process briefly to a rough paste. Tip everything into a bowl. Add the beaten egg and mix thoroughly. With floured hands, form the mixture into 16 small balls and flatten them slightly.

4 Lightly oil a baking sheet and place the ta'amia on it. Sprinkle or brush with olive oil, and bake in the preheated oven for 20 minutes, turning from time to time, until golden. Serve the ta'amia warm with yoghurt on the side.

Variation: if you are in a hurry, the ta'amia can be shallow fried in olive oil instead of baked. Whether baked or fried, they are very appetizing if you serve them sprinkled with dukkah (see page 150).

Note: White haricot beans could be used in place of the butter beans. All pulses are excellent food for diabetics because they are digested slowly, very gradually absorbed into the bloodstream as glucose and thus needing very small quantities of insulin. A regular intake of pulses may help to improve long-term blood glucose control.

48% carbohydrate, GL:

Ta'amia is the Egyptian name for falafel, the deep fried chickpea snack so beloved throughout the Middle East. My version is a little lighter, being baked in the oven rather than deep fried. The butter beans make a refreshing change from the ubiquitous chickpeas. In Egypt dried broad beans (ful) would be used, but these have a very high GI at 113, whereas butter beans are 44.

Per Serving:
Calories (kcal) 186
Protein (g) 8.6
Carbohydrates (g) 18.8
Total Sugars (g) 0.7
Dietary Fibre (g) 4.9
Fat (g) 8.8
Saturated Fat (g) 1.5

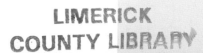

Oatcakes are everywhere these days, and it is easy to buy them ready-made. However, it's more satisfying to make your own. These are made with olive oil rather than the palm oil usually used in commercial oatcakes, and this gives them a lovely flavour and crisp texture. They are suitable for breakfast, as a snack with any of the dips on the preceding pages, or just on their own at any time. This recipe makes quite a lot of oatcakes, but can successfully be halved.

Per Serving:
Calories (kcal) 82.7
Protein (g) 1.8
Carbohydrates (g) 9.1
Total Sugars (g) 0.2
Dietary Fibre (g) 1.2
Fat (g) 4.7
Saturated Fat (g) 0.7

scottish oatcakes

Makes 30 oatcakes **Time taken:** 45 minutes

400g/14 oz (5 cups) rolled oats
1/2 tsp Sea salt
1 tsp Baking powder
120ml/4 fl oz (1/2 cup) Extra virgin olive oil
6 fl oz (175 ml) Hot water

1 Preheat the oven to 150°C/300°F/Gas Mark 2. Spray two baking trays with olive oil spray or wipe with a piece of kitchen paper dipped in olive oil.

2 Put the rolled oats in the food processor and process until quite finely chopped. Add the salt and baking powder. Pour in the olive oil and process briefly, then add the water, and process until a soft dough is formed (you may not need all the water, so go easy). Turn out onto a floured surface and roll out to a thickness of about 2-3mm/⅛ inch. Cut out circles of the dough with a 8cm/3 inch cutter, lift each oatcake off the surface with a palette knife (as they are a little fragile) and place on the baking trays.

3 Bake in the preheated oven for 30 minutes, then cool on a wire rack and store in an airtight tin.

Note: If you don't have rolled oats, porridge oats will do, as they are going to be ground up in any case. I keep the mixture fairly coarse but if you prefer finer oatcakes, process for a little longer.

42% carbohydrate, GL: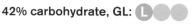

quick soya dhosas

Serves 4 **Time taken:** 45 minutes

110g/4 oz (³/₄ cup) Brown rice flour
45g/1¹/₂ oz (¹/₄ cup) Chickpea (gram) flour
45g/1¹/₂ oz (¹/₄ cup) Soya flour
Sea salt to taste
1 tsp Bicarbonate of soda
1 tsp Coconut oil for frying

1 Mix together the rice flour, chickpea flour, soya flour and salt with approx. 225ml/
8 fl oz/1 cup of water to make a thin batter. Set aside for 30 minutes.

2 When ready to make the dhosas, sprinkle the bicarbonate of soda on the batter and
mix gently.

3 Heat a non-stick pan or tava (a flat or slightly concave hotplate with no sides, thus
making the dhosas easier to turn), and grease it lightly with coconut oil. When hot, pour
one quarter of the batter on the pan and spread it using a circular motion to make a thin
dhosa. As it cooks, pour a little oil around the edge. Continue cooking until it is cooked
through without turning over. When crispy, fold over. Repeat with the remaining batter to
make three more dhosas.

4 Serve hot with the chutney of your choice.

**Note: As well as helping to control blood sugar levels, soya flour is a good source
of protein and vitamin B12.**

Traditional dhosas are large spongy pancakes made from dahl and rice flour, fermented overnight and usually eaten for breakfast in Southern India. I have experimented with them but find that, not only do they take a long time, but also their glycaemic load is just too high. So try these instant Indian pancakes when you want a healthy snack which does not raise your blood sugar levels rapidly. This mixture doesn't need to be fermented overnight. Serve hot, with Coconut Chutney (see page 146).

Per Serving:
Calories (kcal) 192.1
Protein (g) 7.5
Carbohydrates (g) 31.1
Total Sugars (g) 0.6
Dietary Fibre (g) 4.9
Fat (g) 5.2
Saturated Fat (g) 1.8

62% carbohydrate, GL:

.

This snack, known as Pan de Higos, is traditionally made and served at Christmas time. It contains some chocolate, but this is mitigated by the large quantity of nuts, so the overall effect is a reasonable GL. Cut into thin slices, these fig rolls are good to serve after dinner with a cup of tea or coffee.

Per Serving:
Calories (kcal) 248.0
Protein (g) 6.0
Carbohydrates (g) 21.6
Total Sugars (g) 13.3
Dietary Fibre (g) 5.9
Fat (g) 17.1
Saturated Fat (g) 2.0

spanish fig rolls

Makes 3 rolls (4 servings per roll) **Time taken:** 30 minutes

150g/5^1/$_2$ oz (^{3}/$_4$ cup) Hazelnuts
150g/5^1/$_2$ oz (^{3}/$_4$ cup) Almonds
250g/9 oz (1^1/$_4$ cups) Dried figs
1 tsp Cinnamon
^{1}/$_2$ tsp Aniseed or fennel seed, ground
^{1}/$_4$ tsp Ground cloves
^{1}/$_2$ tsp White pepper
1 tbsp Lemon zest, finely grated
45g/1^1/$_2$ oz Dark chocolate (at least 70% cocoa solids), melted
Apple juice
45g/1^1/$_2$ oz Sesame seeds, lightly toasted in a dry pan

1 Finely chop the hazelnuts and almonds, either by hand or in the food processor. Place in a large bowl. Cut the tough stalks off the figs, chop finely and add to the nuts, together with the aniseed or fennel seed, cloves, pepper and lemon zest. Add the melted chocolate and just enough apple juice to moisten the mixture slightly. It should be quite stiff. Mix well with your hands. Form the mixture into three large balls, then roll these into cylinders about 15cm/6 inches long. Roll them in the toasted sesame seeds, then leave to dry for a few hours before wrapping individually in plastic wrap. Store in tightly closed tins or in the fridge – they keep very well. To serve, cut each roll into small slices with a sharp knife.

Note: Everybody knows about the laxative effect of figs – this is due to a substance they contain called mucin which has a soothing and gently cleansing effect on the intestines. They are also a good source of iron and an excellent non-dairy source of calcium.

33% carbohydrate, GL: ●Ⓜ●

chocolate petits fours

Makes 20 **Time taken:** 50 minutes

100g/3¹/₂ oz Dark chocolate – at least 70% cocoa solids
3 tbsp Milk or dairy-free alternative
15g/¹/₂ oz (1 tbsp) Dried cranberries
30g/1 oz (2 tbsp) Dried apricots, chopped
45g/1¹/₂ oz (3 tbsp) Blanched almonds, roughly chopped
45g/1¹/₂ oz (3 tbsp) Pecans, roughly chopped
5 Oatcakes, crumbled (see page 56)
2 tsp Flaked almonds

1 Break the chocolate into small pieces and place in a heavy based pan. Add the milk and heat gently, stirring occasionally, until the chocolate has melted. Remove from the heat and stir until smooth and thoroughly blended.

2 Add the cranberries, apricots, almonds, pecans and crumbled oatcakes and stir until lightly coated with chocolate.

3 Spoon into petit four paper cases, or place teaspoonfuls onto non-stick baking paper. Leave for at least half an hour, or until the mixture has set, then refrigerate. Sprinkle with flaked almonds before serving.

Note: I have made this successfully for a celiac guest using Doves Farm gluten-free savoury biscuits in place of oatcakes.

This is a treat for times of celebration.
Dark chocolate is full of antioxidants and it is quite acceptable to include a little really good quality dark chocolate in a diabetic-friendly diet.
The secret is to eat small portions – as you will note, the glycaemic load of this recipe is low if you only eat one.

Per Serving:
Calories (kcal) 77.8
Protein (g) 1.4
Carbohydrates (g) 6.7
Total Sugars (g) 3.2
Dietary Fibre (g) 1.3
Fat (g) 5.3
Saturated Fat (g) 1.3

34% carbohydrate, GL: ●○○

These relatively healthy bars are useful for a mid-morning snack if you have had a protein breakfast, or a good way to bring up your blood sugar before or after exercise. Take one with you when you go for a walk so you have something to keep you going.

oat, apple and nut snack bars

Makes 16 bars **Time taken:** 40 minutes

200g/7 oz (2 2/3 cups) Jumbo oats
30g/1 oz (1/3 cup) Flax seed
125g/4 1/2 oz (2/3 cup) Mixed nuts
90g/3 oz (1/2 cup) Dried apples, chopped
2 medium Bananas, mashed
1 Free-range egg, lightly beaten
90ml/3 fl oz (1/3 cup) Extra virgin olive oil
2 tsp Cinnamon
2 tbsp Honey

1 Preheat the oven to 180°C/350°F/gas 4. Line a 23 x 30cm/9 x 12 inch baking tray with baking parchment.

2 Combine all the dry ingredients in a large bowl and mix well.

3 Add the mashed bananas, beaten egg, olive oil and honey, and mix well until blended and the mixture is sticky.

4 Press into the prepared baking tray and bake for 20 minutes until the mixture is golden brown. Cool in the pan, and then, using a sharp knife, cut into 16 bars. Stored in an airtight tin, these bars should keep for at least 3 days.

Note: Like many of the recipes in this book, these bars contain cinnamon, which has been shown to lower blood sugar in people with Type 2 diabetes. Half a teaspoon per day appears to be the optimum amount, which should be quite easy to achieve.

Per Serving:
Calories (kcal) 197.9
Protein (g) 3.9
Carbohydrates (g) 20.1
Total Sugars (g) 7
Dietary Fibre (g) 3.3
Fat (g) 12.3
Saturated Fat (g) 1.5

39% carbohydrate, GL: ● M ●

soups and light meals

harira

Harira is a hearty Moroccan soup eaten at evening during Ramadan. There are infinite variations, of course, so this recipe is only a guide. It makes a large quantity, but could quite easily be halved. A light, carbohydrate-free thickening is provided by eggs beaten with lemon, much like the Greek avgolemono.

Serves 8 Time taken: 15 minutes

1 tbsp Extra virgin olive oil
225g/8 oz (¹/₂ pound) Diced lamb
2 large Onions, peeled and chopped
2 Celery sticks, including leaves, chopped
6 tbsp Chopped flat leaf parsley
¹/₂ tsp Freshly ground black pepper
1 tsp Turmeric
1 tsp Ground cinnamon
¹/₄ tsp Ground ginger
90g/3 oz (¹/₂ cup) Lentils
900g/2 lbs Tomatoes, peeled and seeded
Leaves from 2-3 sprigs of fresh coriander
60g/2 oz (¹/₃ cup) Vermicelli noodles
2 Free-range eggs
2 tsp Lemon juice

1 Heat the oil in a large deep pan over medium heat, then add the diced lamb, onions, celery, parsley, pepper, turmeric, cinnamon and ginger. Cook, stirring for about 15 minutes until the ingredients are well browned. Add the lentils along with about 1.4 litres/2¹/₂ pts/7 cups of water. Stir, partially cover the pan, and simmer for 1¹/₂ hours.

2 Purée the tomatoes in a food processor and add to the pot along with the coriander leaves, then simmer for another 15 minutes. Bring the soup to the boil and add the vermicelli, broken into 2.5cm/1" pieces. Reduce the heat and cook for 2-3 minutes more.

3 To thicken the soup, beat the eggs with the lemon juice. Remove the soup from the stove, and stir the egg mixture into it off the heat. Serve at once in heated bowls.

Variations: chicken can be used in place of lamb, and any sort of dried beans, soaked overnight, could replace the lentils. For a spicy kick, 2 teaspoons of harissa (see page 147) could be stirred in with the eggs and lemon juice.

Note: Vermicelli has a modest GI of 35, and because only very little is used per person, it should not have much glycaemic effect.

Per Serving:
Calories (kcal) 195.1
Protein (g) 12.5
Carbohydrates (g) 21.6
Total Sugars (g) 5.5
Dietary Fibre (g) 4.7
Fat (g) 7.1
Saturated Fat (g) 1.8

43% carbohydrate, GL:

beetroot and red cabbage soup

Serves 4 **Time taken:** 1 hour

2 tbsp Extra virgin olive oil
1 Red onion, peeled and finely chopped
2 Garlic cloves, peeled and finely chopped
340g/12 oz Red cabbage, finely shredded
450g/1 lb Raw beetroot, trimmed, peeled and cut into 1cm/1/2" dice
1 large Eating apple, peeled and cut into 1cm/1/2" dice
100ml/3¹/₂ fl oz (¹/₂ cup) Red wine, dry cider or apple juice
600ml/18 fl oz (3 cups) Home-made chicken or vegetable stock
1 Bay leaf
2 Sprigs of fresh thyme
Sea salt and freshly ground black pepper
To serve: Natural live yoghurt
Snipped chives

1 Heat the olive oil in a large saucepan over medium heat and sauté the onion and garlic until they start to colour, stirring occasionally. Add the red cabbage, beetroot and apple, stir well and cook for five minutes to soften. Add the cider or apple juice and turn the heat up to reduce the liquid until it is syrupy, then add the stock, herbs and seasoning, bring to the boil, cover and simmer over low heat for 35-45 minutes until the beetroot is tender. Remove the bay leaf and thyme sprigs.

2 Serve with a spoonful of yoghurt in each bowl, and top with a sprinkling of snipped chives.

Note: This soup is very heart-healthy. Beetroot contains folate which helps to reduce risk of heart disease by reducing homocysteine, a toxic by-product of protein metabolism; and red cabbage supplies the antioxidant lycopene. Research has found that higher intakes of lycopene are associated with lower levels of heart disease, especially in men.

This is a vaguely Russian-inspired, beautifully coloured and very tasty soup. One of my nutritional therapist colleagues commented to me that this was a fabulous way to encourage her patients to eat more beetroot, which we know to be very nutritious.

Per Serving:
Calories (kcal) 165.6
Protein (g) 5.1
Carbohydrates (g) 28.1
Total Sugars (g) 17.3
Dietary Fibre (g) 6.2
Fat (g) 4.5
Saturated Fat (g) 0.7

62% carbohydrate, GL: ● Ⓜ ●

barley and saffron soup

This soup is substantial and filling but moderate GL at the same time. It's a lovely colour, too, from the sweet potato, carrots and saffron. If you don't have saffron, substitute half a teaspoon of turmeric. Although it doesn't have the delicate taste of saffron, it is a good alternative and has anti-inflammatory properties.

Serves 4 Time taken: 1 hour

1 tbsp Extra virgin olive oil
2 Onions, finely chopped
2 sticks Celery, finely chopped
1.4 litres/2³/₄ pts (7 cups) Vegetable stock
90g/3 oz (1 cup) Pearl barley
Large pinch of saffron threads
Sprig of fresh thyme
100g/3¹/₂ oz (1 cup) Sweet potato, peeled and diced
2 Medium carrots, diced
Freshly ground black pepper
1 tbsp Tamari sauce

1 Heat the oil in a large saucepan and gently sauté the onion and celery over low heat until soft. Add the stock, barley, saffron and thyme, bring to the boil and simmer over low heat for 30 minutes. Add the sweet potato and carrot and cook for another 20 minutes, or until the barley and vegetables are tender.

2 Season to taste with pepper, add the tamari, simmer for a further minute or two and serve in hot bowls.

Note: Pearl barley has a relatively low GI. The fibre content of barley accounts for its ability to lower cholesterol and glucose, and the beta-glucans it contains may also reduce appetite by slowing down emptying of the stomach and stabilising blood sugar.

Per Serving:
Calories (kcal) 144.4
Protein (g) 4.1
Carbohydrates (g) 23.1
Total Sugars (g) 7.2
Dietary Fibre (g) 4.5
Fat (g) 4.4
Saturated Fat (g) 0.5

62% carbohydrate, GL: ● Ⓜ ●

peruvian quinoa soup

Serves 4 Time taken: 25 minutes

1 tbsp Extra virgin olive oil
60g/2 oz (¹/₃ cup) Quinoa, rinsed and drained
1 Carrot, diced
1 stick Celery, diced
2 tbsp Finely chopped onions
¹/₂ Green pepper, diced
2 Garlic cloves, crushed
900ml/1¹/₂ pints (1 quart) Good home-made chicken stock
2 large Tomatoes, finely chopped
60g/2 oz (¹/₂ cup) Green cabbage, finely shredded
Sea salt and freshly ground black pepper
Freshly chopped parsley to garnish

1 Heat the oil in a large saucepan; add the quinoa, carrot, celery, onion, pepper and garlic and fry, stirring, until browned.

2 Add the stock and tomatoes, mix well and bring to the boil. Reduce the heat and simmer for 15-20 minutes. Then add the cabbage and continue cooking for another 6-8 minutes, until the cabbage is just cooked and the quinoa is tender.

3 Season with salt and pepper and garnish with parsley. Serve hot.

Note: Quinoa is an excellent source of minerals, especially magnesium and calcium (46mg and 58mg respectively per portion in this soup). It has an excellent protein profile too. Although it doesn't appear in the 2002 GI list, it was subsequently tested and found to have a GI of 51, which is considered low.

This is an approximation of the delicious quinoa soup we were served when I was hiking the Inca Trail in Peru. I bought some red quinoa while I was there and have used that to make this soup often. You can add some pieces of cooked chicken to increase protein and make it more substantial.

Per Serving:
Calories (kcal) 139.6
Protein (g) 4.3
Carbohydrates (g) 19.5
Total Sugars (g) 4.9
Dietary Fibre (g) 3.9
Fat (g) 5.2
Saturated Fat (g) 0.6

55% carbohydrate, GL:

provençal tomato soup with basil and goat's cheese dumplings

This soup is very simple, and only worth making when you can get really flavourful sun-ripened tomatoes, preferably home-grown, so it's best kept for the summer months.

Serves 4 Time taken: 1 hour 15 minutes

900g/2 lb Really ripe tomatoes
3 Garlic cloves, whole
1 litre/1³/₄ pts (4¹/₃ cups) Vegetable stock
1 large Orange, juice only
Sea salt and freshly ground black pepper
For the dumplings
Bunch of fresh basil
75g/2¹/₂ oz (5 tbsp) Mascarpone
75g/2¹/₂ oz (¹/₂ cup) Soft goat's cheese

1 Preheat the oven to 180°C/350°F/Gas Mark 4. Place the whole tomatoes and whole garlic in a roasting tin and roast for about an hour, until the tomatoes split.

2 Take out of the oven and leave to cool a little. Then pop the garlic cloves out of their skins and put in the blender with the tomatoes and enough of the stock to make a purée. Pass through a fine sieve into a clean pan and add the rest of the stock. Add the orange juice and seasoning, and reheat to serve.

3 For the dumplings, chop the basil, and mix with the mascarpone and goat's cheese in a bowl. Float a spoonful of this mixture in each bowl before serving.

Note: The miracle nutrient in tomatoes is lycopene, a powerful antioxidant that seems to protect against heart disease and cancer. It appears to protect against heart disease by deactivating free radicals that damage LDL cholesterol. Damaged LDL can block blood vessels, thus leading to heart attacks.

Per Serving:
Calories (kcal) 212.8
Protein (g) 8.2
Carbohydrates (g) 18.6
Total Sugars (g) 11
Dietary Fibre (g) 3.4
Fat (g) 12.6
Saturated Fat (g) 7.5

34% carbohydrate, GL: M

sweet potato miso soup

Serves 4 Time taken: 20 minutes

1.8 litres/3^{1}/$_{4}$ pints (8 cups) Vegetable stock
675g/1^{1}/$_{2}$ lbs Sweet potatoes, cut into thin slices and then into bite-sized pieces
50ml/2 fl oz (^{1}/$_{4}$ cup) Sake or dry white wine
60g/1 oz Daikon radish, shredded (optional)
2.5cm/1" (1 inch) piece Fresh ginger root
1^{1}/$_{2}$ tsp Tamari
4 tbsp (^{1}/$_{3}$ cup) Sweet white miso
125g/4^{1}/$_{2}$ oz Tofu, cut into 0.5cm/^{1}/$_{4}$" cubes (half a packet)
2 tbsp Spring onions, finely sliced

1 Put the stock and sweet potatoes into a large saucepan with the sake and daikon, if using. Simmer until the sweet potatoes are barely tender – they should not be falling apart. This may take as little as 5 minutes, but not longer than 10 minutes. The skill in making this soup is to allow the sweet potato to cook but to hold its shape.

2 Peel and grate the ginger, then squeeze the grated ginger with your hand into a small bowl to extract the juice – you need about a teaspoonful. Ladle 300ml/^{1}/$_{2}$ pint/1 cup of the cooking liquid into the bowl with the ginger juice and add the tamari and miso. Leave to stand for 5 minutes, then stir until smooth. Add the miso mixture back into the soup and stir to mix. Add the tofu and sliced spring onions to the pot and reheat briefly. Ladle into 4 heated soup bowls and serve immediately.

Note: Daikon is a variety of radish also known as Japanese or Chinese radish. They are white with a milder flavour than the small red radish, and much larger – usually 1-5lbs. Daikon can be eaten raw in salad, pickled, or used in stir fries, soups and stews. They have a pleasant, sweet and zesty flavour with a mild bite.

This Japanese soup uses the sweet white miso rather than the more familiar dark brown miso. It is available in health food shops, and is supplied by Clearspring Ltd (see Useful Addresses).

Per Serving:
Calories (kcal) 239.6
Protein (g) 11.5
Carbohydrates (g) 38.9
Total Sugars (g) 17.5
Dietary Fibre (g) 8.8
Fat (g) 3.5
Saturated Fat (g) 0.4

63% carbohydrate, GL:

Ribollita means re-boiled in Italian, and this rustic Italian soup tastes even better reheated the next day. My recipe is a quick and easy version of the traditional soup, which would probably contain pancetta and stale bread among other things. If you can't get fresh basil to make the basil oil, use the basil preserved in jars of olive oil available in supermarkets.

Per Serving:
Calories (kcal) 378.2
Protein (g) 13.7
Carbohydrates (g) 40.3
Total Sugars (g) 4.2
Dietary Fibre (g) 9.6
Fat (g) 18.8
Saturated Fat (g) 2.6

ribollita with basil oil

Serves 4 Time taken: 1¹/₂ hours or 30 minutes if using canned beans

200g/7 oz (1 cup) Dried white beans, such as cannellini beans or white haricot beans, or use two 400g/14 oz cans
1 tbsp Extra virgin olive oil
3 Garlic cloves crushed
1 Onion, peeled and finely chopped
2 Carrots, finely sliced
600ml/1 pt (2¹/₂ cups) Vegetable stock
1 tbsp Tomato purée
200g/14 oz Savoy cabbage, quartered, cored and shredded
Sea salt and freshly ground black pepper
For the basil oil: A generous handful of fresh basil
60ml/2 fl oz (¹/₄ cup) Extra virgin olive oil
Pinch of salt
¹/₂ Garlic clove

1 If using dried beans, you will need to soak them overnight in cold water. Next day, drain the beans and boil them until tender, about 45 minutes to 1 hour. Drain, reserving 8 fl oz/1 cup of the cooking liquid. If using canned beans, simply drain and rinse, then proceed with the recipe. Put half the beans into a blender and whizz together with the reserved cooking liquid, or (if you are using canned beans) with the same amount of water, to make a smooth purée.

2 Heat the olive oil in a large pan and cook the garlic, onion and carrots for 5 minutes over medium heat until starting to soften, stirring occasionally.

3 Add the puréed and whole beans, stock and tomato purée and bring to a simmer, stirring from time to time. Add the cabbage and cook for a further 6-8 minutes, until the cabbage is just tender. Season to taste.

4 Meanwhile, make the basil oil: whizz the basil, oil, salt and garlic in a blender until smooth, and leave to stand so that it settles and loses its milky texture.

5 Serve the soup with a spoonful of basil oil on each serving.

Note: A particularly good source of soluble fibre, haricot beans (of which cannellini beans are a variety) also contain more calcium and magnesium than other varieties (166mg and 92mg respectively per serving of this soup). There's also a good range of antioxidants in this soup from all the different vegetables.

43% carbohydrate, GL:

fish and watercress soup with ginger

Serves 4 Time taken: 40 minutes

15g/$^1/_2$ oz Dried shiitake mushrooms
125ml/4 fl oz ($^1/_2$ cup) Hot water
2 tsp Extra virgin olive oil
1 tsp Oriental (toasted) sesame oil
2 Spring onions, finely chopped
2 Garlic cloves, peeled and finely chopped
2.5 cm/1" (1 inch) piece Root ginger, peeled and finely chopped
750ml/1$^1/_4$ pt (3$^1/_4$ cups) Chicken stock
2 tbsp Thai fish sauce
1 tbsp Dry sherry (optional)
1 tbsp Tamari
225g/8 oz ($^1/_2$ pound) White fish, such as hoki, cut into 2 cm/$^3/_4$" cubes
3 bunches Watercress, washed and chopped

1 Soak the mushrooms in a little hot water until softened, about 20 minutes. Drain them, reserving the soaking liquid. Squeeze out excess moisture. Thinly slice the mushroom caps and discard the stems.

2 Heat the olive and sesame oils in a heavy large saucepan over medium heat.
Add the spring onions, garlic and ginger and sauté until just tender, about 3 minutes.
Add the sliced mushrooms and sauté until mushrooms are tender, about 3 minutes.
Add the chicken stock, the mushroom soaking liquid, Thai fish sauce, sherry (if using) and tamari sauce. Bring to the boil. Stir in the fish and boil until the fish is just cooked through, about 2 minutes. Add the watercress and cook for another minute – no longer or the watercress will lose its bright green colour. Serve immediately in hot bowls.

Note: Watercress is a superfood and should be eaten regularly. It is a particularly good vegetable source of calcium, which is important for bones, healthy muscles and nerves, and the beta carotenes it contains are protective of eye health. The peppery taste is caused by a mustard oil which is a powerful natural antibiotic.

The inspiration for this soup is South East Asian.

Per Serving:
Calories (kcal) 157.7
Protein (g) 12.4
Carbohydrates (g) 5.4
Total Sugars (g) 1.0
Dietary Fibre (g) 1.6
Fat (g) 9.0
Saturated Fat (g) 1.2

14% carbohydrate, GL: L ● ●

chilled avocado soup

Fashions for chilled soups come and go, but this Mexican soup is one that cannot fail to please, especially before a hot spicy main dish.
Try to find the dark-skinned Californian Hass avocados for this,
as they are the creamiest variety, and use home-made vegetable stock for the best flavour.

Serves 4 Time taken: 15 minutes

1 tbsp Lemon juice
1 tbsp Lime juice
2 Spring onions, trimmed
900ml/1¹/₂ pts (3³/₄ cups) Vegetable stock, preferably home- made
1 tbsp Fresh mint leaves
¹/₂ tsp Ground cumin
Pinch of cayenne pepper
Sea salt and freshly ground black pepper to taste
3 large Ripe Hass avocados, peeled, stones removed, cut into chunks
2 tbsp Finely chopped red pepper, for garnish

1 Put the lemon and lime juices, spring onions, vegetable stock, mint, spices and seasoning in the blender and blend until smooth. Add the avocados and blend again until just creamy. Pour into a bowl or jug, cover and refrigerate.

2 Serve in chilled bowls, garnished with the finely chopped red pepper.

Note: Avocados have an excellent nutritional profile. They are a very good source of soluble fibre and a rich source of potassium. This soup delivers 715mg of potassium in each serving, so is ideal for those with high blood pressure. Because avocados turn brown on exposure to the air, this soup should be served within a couple of hours of blending.

Per Serving:
Calories (kcal) 253
Protein (g) 3.8
Carbohydrates (g) 17.8
Total Sugars (g) 3.6
Dietary Fibre (g) 10.4
Fat (g) 20.6
Saturated Fat (g) 2.8

26% carbohydrate, GL: **L** ● ●

arame with baked vegetables

Serves 3 Time taken: 50 minutes

15 g/¹/₂ oz Arame (a large handful)
2 medium Onions, peeled and quartered
2 medium Carrots, peeled unless organic, and cut into chunks
2 Courgettes, thickly sliced
2 Red peppers, deseeded and cut into pieces
110g/4 oz (1 cup) Mushrooms, cut in half if large
2 Garlic cloves, peeled and finely chopped
2 tbsp Extra virgin olive oil
1 tbsp Concentrated apple juice
To serve: 1 tbsp Tamari
2 tbsp Coriander leaves, roughly chopped

1 Preheat the oven to 190°C/375°F/gas 5.

2 Rinse the arame under cold water. Place it in a bowl and cover with cold water. Soak for 10 minutes, then rinse again and drain well.

3 Place the drained arame and all the other ingredients (except the tamari and coriander) in a large ovenproof casserole, and mix well. Add about 6 tablespoons of boiling water, just enough to moisten. Cover with a lid and bake until the vegetables are tender (approximately 35-40 minutes). Sprinkle with the tamari sauce, garnish with the chopped coriander and serve hot.

Variation: you can use any vegetables for this dish, according to what's in season. For example, in winter you might like to try squash and beetroot in place of the courgettes and peppers.

Note: Like other seaweeds, arame contains all of the minerals required by human beings, including calcium, sodium, magnesium, potassium, iodine, iron, and zinc. In addition, there are many trace elements in seaweeds. Oriental medicine has long recognised that sea vegetables contribute to the health of the endocrine and nervous systems. In recent decades, medical researchers have discovered that a diet that includes sea vegetables reduces the risk of some diseases, including diabetes.

Arame is a mildly flavoured seaweed that has been precooked and sliced finely. It is therefore an ideal food with which to start an exploration of sea vegetables. It expands hugely when soaked and cooked, so although a handful might seem like a small amount, it will swell dramatically.

Per Serving:
Calories (kcal) 221.4
Protein (g) 3.0
Carbohydrates (g) 21.2
Total Sugars (g) 13.1
Dietary Fibre (g) 3.3
Fat (g) 15.2
Saturated Fat (g) 2.0

37% carbohydrate, GL: M

These little cakes are a healthy improvement on the more usual courgette fritters, which are coated in batter and deep-fried.

greek courgette cakes

Serves 6 **Time taken:** 50 minutes

450g/1lb Courgettes
Sea salt
6 Spring onions, finely chopped
2 Free-range eggs, lightly beaten
100g/3^1/2 oz (^{1}/2 cup) Feta cheese, crumbled
60g/2 oz (^{3}/4 cup) Wholemeal, rye or gluten-free breadcrumbs
1 handful Fresh mint, finely chopped
^{1}/2 tsp Nutmeg
Freshly ground black pepper
110g/4 oz (^{2}/3 cup) Cornmeal or polenta
2 tbsp Extra virgin olive oil
Lemon wedges, to serve

1 Grate the courgettes, sprinkle with salt and place in a colander to drain off moisture for 30 minutes.

2 Rinse the courgettes well and squeeze with your hands to remove any remaining liquid. Dry on kitchen paper.

3 Mix the courgettes with the onions, eggs, feta, breadcrumbs, mint and nutmeg. Season to taste with pepper (you should not need salt as the feta is salty). Form into 16 small cakes, and roll in the polenta until coated all over.

4 Heat the olive oil in a roomy frying pan over medium high heat. Fry the courgette cakes for about 3 minutes on each side until crisp and golden. Drain on kitchen paper and serve hot with lemon wedges.

Note: **Courgettes are easy to digest, mildly laxative and diuretic. They are also useful for the relief of bladder and kidney infections, and are recommended for people with diabetes. Note that this recipe is quite high in sodium owing to the feta and the salting of the courgettes. You could skip salting the courgettes, but you may find the mixture is too wet if you do.**

Per Serving:
Calories (kcal) 223.6
Protein (g) 9.4
Carbohydrates (g) 24.3
Total Sugars (g) 2.5
Dietary Fibre (g) 4.3
Fat (g) 10.1
Saturated Fat (g) 3.1

43% carbohydrate, GL: ● Ⓜ ●

kerala vegetable curry

Serves 4 Time taken: 55 minutes

2 tbsp Coconut oil
1 tsp Mustard seeds
2 Green chillies, deseeded and chopped
1 small bunch Curry leaves (only if fresh)
2 Onions, peeled and chopped
1/2 tsp Ground coriander
1 tsp Cumin seeds
1/2 tsp Garam masala (see page 144)
1/4 tsp Turmeric
1/4 tsp Chilli powder
6 Tomatoes, peeled and chopped
2 Sweet potatoes, peeled
1 medium Aubergine
200ml/7 fl oz (3/4 cup) Coconut milk
100g/31/2 oz (1 cup) French beans
100g/31/2 oz (1 cup) Peas, frozen or fresh podded
100g/31/2 oz (1 cup) Okra
Sea salt and freshly ground black pepper

1 Heat the coconut oil in a pan and fry the mustard seeds for 2-3 minutes or until they start to pop.

2 Add the chillies, curry leaves, onions, coriander, cumin seeds, garam masala, turmeric and chilli powder. Stir and cook until the onion is soft, then add the chopped tomatoes.

3 Chop the sweet potatoes and aubergine into small cubes and add to the sauce. Pour in the coconut milk and cook until the sweet potato is soft and cooked through. Add the beans, fresh peas and okra, season and cook for another 6-7 minutes or until the vegetables are tender (if using frozen peas, hold them back until a couple of minutes before serving).

Note: The sweet potato in this curry is a diabetic-friendly food. It is an excellent source of beta-carotene, a very good source of vitamin C and manganese, and a good source of copper, dietary fibre, vitamin B6, potassium and iron. It has recently been classified as an 'antidiabetic' food because in some recent animal studies sweet potato was shown to help stabilise blood glucose levels and lower insulin resistance.

49% carbohydrate, GL: ● M ●

Serve this Southern Indian curry with sweet cinnamon rice (page 102) and a raita of your choice. Curry leaves can be found in Asian shops, but only use them if fresh, as the dried ones have little flavour. If you find fresh curry leaves, they can be frozen: just take the leaves off the stalk and freeze in a sealed bag.

Per Serving:
Calories (kcal) 267.9
Protein (g) 7.4
Carbohydrates (g) 35.1
Total Sugars (g) 13.1
Dietary Fibre (g) 7.4
Fat (g) 12.9
Saturated Fat (g) 10.5

mediterranean roasted vegetables with beans

Serves 4 **Time taken:** 45 minutes

285g/10 oz (3 cups) Cherry tomatoes
2 small Red peppers, de-seeded and sliced
2 small Green peppers, de-seeded and sliced
2 small Onions, peeled and sliced into 2.5cm/1" squares
2 medium Courgettes
110g/4 oz Fennel, cut into 2.5cm/1" slices
2 tbsp Extra virgin olive oil
2 Garlic cloves, peeled and crushed
2 tbsp Lemon juice
2 tbsp Fresh basil leaves, chopped
Black pepper to taste
60g/2 oz (4 tbsp) Black olives
110g/4 oz (1 cup) Feta cheese, cut into cubes
450g/1lb Cooked mixed beans, or use canned beans, rinsed and drained
To serve: Torn basil leaves

1 Preheat the oven to 180°C/350°F/gas 4.

2 Arrange the tomatoes, peppers, onion, courgettes and fennel in a roasting tin. Mix together the olive oil, garlic, lemon juice and basil leaves and sprinkle over the vegetables. Toss together, season with black pepper, cover with a lid or foil, and roast for about 30 minutes until the vegetables look a little toasted.

3 Remove from the oven, cool to room temperature, then add the olives and feta cheese.

4 Place the beans in a large serving dish. Top with the vegetable mixture and garnish with torn basil leaves.

Note: Beans are an excellent source of vegetarian protein. Of the bean family, soya beans, butter beans and haricot beans appear to have the lowest GI, so any of these would be a good choice.

A substantial dish, best served at room temperature, this needs no accompaniment, except perhaps some green leaves. Note that this dish is high in sodium, due to the feta cheese and olives.

Per Serving:
Calories (kcal) 301.4
Protein (g) 11.2
Carbohydrates (g) 32.0
Total Sugars (g) 8.3
Dietary Fibre (g) 8.8
Fat (g) 15.5
Saturated Fat (g) 5.5

41% carbohydrate, GL: M

tofu and coriander cakes

Serves 4 **Time taken:** 15 minutes

8 Spring onions, roughly chopped
5 cm/2" piece Fresh root ginger, peeled and chopped
Small handful of fresh coriander, chopped
3 Garlic cloves, peeled and chopped
1 tbsp Tamari sauce
250g/9 oz Tofu, drained, rinsed and dried (1 packet)
90g/3 oz (1 cup) Fresh wholemeal, rye or gluten-free breadcrumbs
1 Free-range egg, beaten
Sea salt and freshly ground black pepper
1 tbsp Groundnut oil

1 Put the spring onions, ginger, coriander and garlic into a food processor or blender and process until mixed together but not a homogenised paste. Add the tamari, tofu, breadcrumbs, beaten egg and seasoning, and process until combined.

2 With wet hands, form the mixture into twelve little flat cakes. Preheat the grill.

3 Place the cakes on a lightly oiled grill pan and brush with a little groundnut oil. Grill under high heat for 2-3 minutes on each side until golden.

Note: Tofu purchased in the UK is normally made using calcium sulphate as a coagulant, so it is naturally high in calcium – these cakes deliver 109mg of calcium per portion. Tofu in Japan is more usually coagulated with nigari, which is mostly magnesium chloride, so it will have a different nutritional profile.

I created this recipe while I was looking for tasty ways of using tofu. The inspiration is broadly Oriental, though the use of breadcrumbs is not very authentic.

Per Serving:
Calories (kcal) 183.1
Protein (g) 12.7
Carbohydrates (g) 15.6
Total Sugars (g) 2.4
Dietary Fibre (g) 3.3
Fat (g) 9.4
Saturated Fat (g) 1.7

32% carbohydrate, GL: L ● ●

thai fish cakes with sweet and sour cucumber sauce

Serves 4 **Time taken:** 15 minutes

450g/1 lb White fish, such as coley, skinned and cut into chunks
1 tbsp Thai fish sauce (Nam Pla)
1 tbsp Thai red curry paste
1 Kaffir lime leaf or 1 strip of lime peel, very finely shredded
1 tbsp Chopped fresh coriander
1 Free-range egg
1/2 tsp Sea salt
45g/1 1/2 oz French beans, thinly sliced into rounds
2 tbsp Groundnut oil
For the sauce: 5cm/2" Unpeeled cucumber
2 Spring onions
1 small Carrot
1 Red birdseye chilli, deseeded and thinly sliced
1 tsp Grated fresh ginger root
1 tbsp Soft brown sugar
120ml/4 fl oz (1/2 cup) Rice vinegar or white wine vinegar
1 tsp Tamari
1 tbsp Groundnut oil

This is a recipe for those tasty little fish cakes served in Thai restaurants as an appetizer. They can be made with any sort of white fish and are substantial enough for a light meal, if served with a salad or some green vegetables.

1 Place the fish in a food processor with the fish sauce, curry paste, kaffir lime leaf or lime peel, chopped coriander, egg and salt. Process lightly, until minced but not too smooth, then turn out into a bowl and stir in the sliced green beans. Divide the mixture into 16 pieces, roll each one into a ball and flatten with the palm of your hand into a 6cm/2.5" disk. Put on a plate, cover with clingfilm and refrigerate for at least an hour, until firm.

2 Meanwhile, make the sauce. Place the cucumber, spring onions, carrot, chilli, and ginger in a food processor and whizz until very finely chopped. Transfer the chopped vegetables to a bowl. Next mix the sugar with the vinegar to dissolve it, then pour it over the vegetables along with the tamari and groundnut oil. Mix thoroughly. Serve in small ramekins.

3 Heat the oil in a large frying pan and fry the fish cakes in batches for one minute on each side, until golden brown. Lift out, drain well on kitchen paper, then serve with the dipping sauce.

Per Serving:
Calories (kcal) 303.8
Protein (g) 30.4
Carbohydrates (g) 13.6
Total Sugars (g) 5.5
Dietary Fibre (g) 2.1
Fat (g) 14
Saturated Fat (g) 2.6

18% carbohydrate, GL: L ● ●

meat, poultry and fish

navarin of lamb

Serves 6 **Time taken:** 2 hours

A lovely light French casserole, suitable for spring lamb, this dish depends for its effect on really fresh baby vegetables. But if you can't get fresh peas, frozen ones work very well.

1.5kg/3^1/$_4$ lb Lean lamb, trimmed and cut into 5cm/2" cubes
1 tbsp Plain flour or gluten-free flour, seasoned
2 tbsp Extra virgin olive oil
750ml/1^1/$_4$ pts (3^1/$_4$ cups) Lamb or chicken stock
3 tbsp Tomato paste
4 Sprigs fresh thyme
1 Bay leaf
2 Cloves garlic, peeled and crushed
18 Pearl onions
18 baby Carrots
18 baby Turnips
175g/6oz French beans, topped, tailed and cut in half
225g/8 oz (^{1}/$_2$ pound) Shelled fresh peas or frozen peas

1 Preheat the oven to 180°C/350°F/gas 4.

2 Toss the meat in the seasoned flour. Heat the oil in a frying pan and brown the meat in batches. Transfer to an ovenproof casserole. Pour the stock into the frying pan and bring to the boil, scraping with a wooden spoon. Pour over the meat. Add the tomato paste, thyme, bay leaf and garlic. Bring to a simmer, then cover and put in the preheated oven for one hour.

3 Meanwhile, place the onions in a bowl and pour boiling water over them. Leave for a few minutes, then peel and trim the bases. Trim the turnips and carrots but leave a little green stalk on each one.

4 Take the casserole out of the oven and skim off as much of the fat as you can. Add the onions, carrot and turnips to the lamb and stir gently to mix. Cover and return to the oven for 30-45 minutes, or until the vegetables are tender.

5 Cook the beans and peas in boiling water for a few minutes. If the peas are frozen they will only need a minute or two. Drain and plunge into cold water to set the colour.

6 Just before serving, stir the beans and peas into the casserole and reheat briefly. Taste for seasoning and serve hot.

Note: Lamb used to be considered a fatty meat, but lean lamb, particularly leg, can contain as little as 2.2g fat per 100g.

Per Serving:
Calories (kcal) 478.7
Protein (g) 56.4
Carbohydrates (g) 26.1
Total Sugars (g) 9.1
Dietary Fibre (g) 7.4
Fat (g) 15.6
Saturated Fat (g) 4.4

22% carbohydrate, GL:

tagine of lamb with apricots and preserved lemons

Serves 6 **Time taken:** 1 hour 35 minutes

2 tbsp Extra virgin olive oil
1.35kg/3 lbs Lean leg of lamb, trimmed and cut into 5cm/2" cubes
2 large Onions, peeled and finely chopped
4 Garlic cloves, peeled and finely chopped
1 tsp Ground ginger
1 tsp Ground cumin
1 tsp Ground turmeric
Freshly ground black pepper
2 Preserved lemons or one home-preserved lemon
12 Unsulphured dried apricots, soaked in water
2 tbsp Flat leaf parsley, roughly chopped
2 tbsp Fresh coriander, roughly chopped

1 Heat the olive oil in a heavy pan and brown the lamb on all sides. Add the onions, stir and cook for a minute or two, then add the garlic and spices. Season with pepper. Add enough water to cover the mixture, cover the pan and turn the heat to very low. Cook for at least an hour, stirring from time to time, or until the meat is tender when pierced with a fork. It may need a little longer.

2 Prepare the preserved lemons: discard the flesh and cut the rind into shreds. Take the lid off the tagine and add the apricots and lemon. Cook for another 20-30 minutes with the lid off, to allow the juices to reduce. Check for seasoning – you should not need to add salt as the lemons are quite salty. Serve sprinkled with the chopped herbs.

Note: I have used lean leg of lamb here, but this tagine can also be made with a cheaper, fattier cut of lamb such as shoulder. It would need to cook for longer than specified in the recipe to become really tender. If using a fattier cut, make the tagine in advance, leave to cool, then skim the fat off the top and reheat until piping hot. This dish would normally be made with saffron, but I have replaced it with turmeric owing to its anti-inflammatory, antioxidant properties. Note that this recipe is fairly high in sodium, from the preserved lemons.

You can buy preserved lemons at large supermarkets, or you can make them yourself (see page 151). If you can't find any preserved lemons, use the peeled rind of a large fresh lemon and chop it with a teaspoon of capers or a handful of pitted green olives to get the briny taste.

Per Serving:
Calories (kcal) 326.7
Protein (g) 39.9
Carbohydrates (g) 11.8
Total Sugars (g) 0.6
Dietary Fibre (g) 0.6
Fat (g) 12.9
Saturated Fat (g) 3.5

15% carbohydrate, GL: L ● ●

This is a Mexican chicken dish using lots of parsley and coriander which gives it what one of my recipe testers described a rather a lurid green colour. Never mind the colour – it tastes delicious.

Per Serving:
Calories (kcal) 542.2
Protein (g) 50.2
Carbohydrates (g) 14.1
Total Sugars (g) 4.7
Dietary Fibre (g) 5.9
Fat (g) 32.3
Saturated Fat (g) 10

pollo verde almendrado

Serves 4 **Time taken:** 1 hour 15 minutes

1 Organic free-range chicken, cut into 12 pieces, or 1.6kg/3^1/$_2$ lbs chicken pieces, skinned
450ml/16 fl oz (2 cups) Fresh chicken stock
1 large Onion, peeled and finely chopped
1 Garlic clove, peeled and finely chopped
60g/2 oz Fresh parsley, chopped
60g/2 oz Fresh coriander, chopped
1 Baby Cos lettuce heart, shredded
100g/3^1/$_2$ oz (1 cup) Ground almonds
1 Green chilli, deseeded and finely chopped
Sea salt and freshly ground black pepper

1 Put the chicken, stock, onion and garlic into a large flameproof casserole or heavy bottomed pan. Bring to the boil, then reduce the heat to a simmer, cover and cook gently until the chicken is tender. This will take about 45 minutes. Lift the chicken out and set aside. Strain the remaining mixture, reserving the onion and the liquid separately.

2 Combine the cooked onion and garlic with the parsley, coriander, shredded lettuce, ground almonds and chilli in the blender. With the motor running, pour in the reserved stock until you get a fairly chunky sauce.

3 Return the chicken pieces to the casserole and pour over the blended sauce. Reheat gently until everything is heated through. Serve with brown rice and green vegetables or salad.

Note: Using almonds for thickening boosts the protein content of a dish, as well as providing a good source of calcium, magnesium and zinc. You could substitute other ground nuts such as hazelnuts or walnuts.

10% carbohydrate, GL: 🅛 ⚪ ⚪

chiang mai chicken curry

Serves 4 **Time taken:** 45 minutes

For the curry paste: 2 tsp Coriander seeds
1 tsp Cumin seeds
3 Cloves
2 Cardamom pods
1 Star anise
5 Dried long red chillies, deseeded, soaked and drained
Pinch of sea salt
3 tbsp Lemongrass, chopped
5cm/2" piece Fresh root ginger, chopped
1 tsp Turmeric
4 Shallots, chopped
6 Garlic cloves, peeled and chopped
For the curry: 1 Organic, free-range chicken, about 1.6kg/3½ lbs
2 Garlic cloves, peeled
2 cm/1" piece Fresh ginger root, peeled
2 tbsp Coconut oil
12 Shallots, peeled
2 tbsp Cashew nuts
2 tbsp Fish sauce
Water or chicken stock, to cover

1 First, dry fry the coriander seeds, star anise, cumin seeds, whole cloves and cardamom pods in a small dry pan until fragrant. When cooled, remove the cardamom seeds and discard the pods. Grind the spices in a pestle and mortar. Combine these with the other curry paste ingredients and mix to a paste either in the mortar or in a food processor.

2 Wash the chicken, joint into 8 pieces and remove the skin. Mash the garlic cloves and ginger to make a paste. In a large pan, heat the coconut oil and fry the garlic and ginger paste until golden. Add the curry paste and chicken and simmer for several minutes, turning frequently. Add the whole shallots and cashew nuts. Season with the fish sauce. Cover with stock or water and simmer for at least 30 minutes, or until the chicken is tender.

Note: The combination of chicken and nuts gives this dish a very high magnesium content (125g per serving). Magnesium is a key mineral for diabetics: and it has been shown that people with low magnesium status are at higher risk of Type 2 diabetes.

20% carbohydrate, GL:

The original of this recipe was given to me years ago by a friend who had lived in Thailand. The chillies specified were unfamiliar to me, and of course the strength and taste of the chillies used can substantially alter a dish. This is not intended to be a very hot curry. Be guided by what chillies are available to you and how hot you like your food. In general, the smaller the chillies the hotter they are, and removing the seeds reduces the heat considerably.

Per Serving:
Calories (kcal) 518.8
Protein (g) 48.9
Carbohydrates (g) 26.9
Total Sugars (g) 4.4
Dietary Fibre (g) 3.1
Fat (g) 24.9
Saturated Fat (g) 10.1

cardamom chicken

Serves 4 **Time taken:** 40 minutes plus overnight standing

1 **Organic free-range chicken (about 1.6kg/3^1/$_2$ lbs)**
2 tsp **Peeled, grated fresh ginger root**
2 tsp **Fresh garlic, finely chopped**
2 tsp **Crushed cardamom seeds**
^{1}/$_2$ tsp **Freshly ground black pepper**
1 **Lime, grated zest and juice**
2 tbsp **Coconut oil**
1 recipe **Labneh made using 600ml/1 pint/2^1/$_2$ cups natural yoghurt (see page 141)**
400g tin (1^1/$_2$ cups) **Coconut milk**
6 large **Mild green chillies**
^{1}/$_2$ bunch **Fresh coriander, chopped**
Sea salt to taste

1 Joint and skin the chicken and put in a dish. Put the ginger, garlic, cardamom and black pepper into the blender and blend to a paste. Add the grated lime zest and spread this over the chicken pieces. Cover the dish and leave to marinate in the fridge overnight.

2 Next day, heat the coconut oil in a large pan and brown the chicken pieces all over. Tip the labneh into the pan, add the coconut milk, stir well and bring to the boil. Now add the whole chillies, having pricked them all over with a fork, and the coriander. Turn the heat down to low, cover and simmer for 20-30 minutes, or until the chicken is tender and cooked through. Taste for seasoning, then add the lime juice before serving.

Note: The combination of ginger, garlic and chillies, so familiar in Asian cooking, delivers a powerful therapeutic punch. Ginger is warming and stimulating, eases digestion and is a natural anti-inflammatory, garlic is a natural antibiotic and chillies stimulate stomach acid, thus killing bacteria.

This delightful fusion of Indian and Thai flavours comes from the Star of India restaurant in Old Brompton Road, London. I have further confused its origins by using the Middle Eastern labneh to make the dish creamier. It involves marinating the chicken overnight, so start the day before you plan to serve the curry. It is worth the wait.

Per Serving:
Calories (kcal) 598.6
Protein (g) 49.4
Carbohydrates (g) 15.7
Total Sugars (g) 2.4
Dietary Fibre (g) 2.8
Fat (g) 38.8
Saturated Fat (g) 27.7

10% carbohydrate, GL: Ⓛ ● ●

turkey mole

Serves 4 Time taken: 1 hour 10 minutes

1 tbsp **Extra virgin olive oil**
4 **Turkey breast fillets**
1 litre/1³/₄ pints (4¹/₃ cups) **Chicken stock**
2 tsp **Dried chillies, crushed**
¹/₄ tsp **Ground cinnamon**
¹/₄ tsp **Ground cloves**
¹/₄ tsp **Roast, ground coriander seed**
¹/₄ tsp **Freshly ground black pepper**
¹/₄ tsp **Star anise, dry roasted and ground**
¹/₂ tsp **Sea salt**
1 large **Onion, peeled and roughly chopped**
2 **Tomatoes, skinned and roughly chopped**
60g/2 oz (4 tbsp) **Ground almonds**
30g/1 oz (2 tbsp) **Raisins**
2 tsp **Sesame seeds**
1 **Garlic clove, peeled and finely chopped**
2 **Corn tortillas, torn into pieces**
30g/1 oz **Dark chocolate**
15g/¹/₂ oz (1 tbsp) **Organic unsalted butter**
Sea salt to taste
To serve: Corn tortillas

1 Preheat the oven to 180°C/350°F/gas 4. Sprinkle the olive oil on the turkey breasts and cook, covered, in a medium hot oven for about 20 minutes until almost cooked. Keep warm. Meanwhile, boil half of the stock together with the crushed chillies and leave to soak for half an hour.

2 Then add the ground cinnamon, cloves, coriander seeds, black pepper, ground star anise, salt, onion, tomatoes, ground almonds, raisins, half of the sesame seeds, garlic and torn tortilla pieces to the stock and chillies. Place in a food processor and purée into a sauce.

3 Melt the butter in a heavy saucepan, add the puréed sauce and simmer for 5 minutes. Add the remainder of the stock and the chocolate and stir until the chocolate is completely melted.

4 Return the turkey to the sauce and simmer for 30 minutes. Season to taste and serve hot with tortillas.

22% carbohydrate, GL:

This is a simplified version of the famous Mexican dish featuring mole – a highly flavoured sauce made from a paste of chillies, chocolate and spices.

Turkey is a good low-fat source of protein, and is especially rich in the amino acid tryptophan, which is needed for the production of the neurotransmitter serotonin. This helps the body to maintain a feeling of wellbeing and combat depression.

Per Serving:
Calories (kcal) 423.1
Protein (g) 33.5
Carbohydrates (g) 23.2
Total Sugars (g) 12.8
Dietary Fibre (g) 5.2
Fat (g) 22.1
Saturated Fat (g) 6.8

seared salmon fillets with spicy soba noodles

Japanese soba noodles, which are made from buckwheat, can be cooked in advance and served at room temperature without losing their texture. The amount of buckwheat in soba varies from 40% to 100% and it gives the noodles their characteristic dark colour and rich, nutty taste. Wasabi and pickled ginger can be obtained from Oriental shops, and increasingly now from supermarkets.

Serves 4 **Time taken:** 40 minutes

4 x 170g/6 oz fillets of wild or organic salmon, skinned
1 tbsp Tamari
$1/2$ tsp Toasted sesame oil
For the noodles: 225g/8 oz ($1/2$ pound) Soba noodles
4 tbsp Tamari
$1/2$ tsp Toasted sesame oil
1 tbsp Groundnut oil
1 tbsp Rice or wine vinegar
1 small Red chilli, deseeded and finely chopped
1 Garlic clove, peeled and finely chopped
2.5cm/1" piece Fresh ginger root, peeled and finely chopped
1 Bunch spring onions, cut into 1cm/$1/2$" slices
110g/4 oz Mangetout peas, topped, tailed and cut into 2.5cm/1" slices
1 Red pepper, deseeded and cut into fine strips
1 tbsp Sesame seeds
Garnish: 2 tsp Wasabi
2 tsp Pickled ginger

1 Put the salmon fillets in a dish. Mix together the tamari and sesame oil and sprinkle over the fillets, turning them so that both sides have come into contact with the marinade. Leave to stand for half an hour.

2 Bring a large pan of water to the boil and cook the soba noodles for 7-8 minutes, until al dente. Drain and refresh in cold water to prevent overcooking.

3 For the sauce, put into a small saucepan the tamari, sesame oil, groundnut oil, rice vinegar, chopped chilli, garlic and ginger. Bring to the boil over medium heat, reduce the heat and simmer for 3-4 minutes to allow the flavours to meld. Set aside.

4 For the vegetables, blanch the mangetout and red pepper strips in boiling water for 2 minutes, drain and refresh in cold water. Toast the sesame seeds in a small dry pan until fragrant.

5 To assemble, drain the noodles well, then toss with the tamari sauce and vegetables. Sprinkle on the toasted sesame seeds.

Per Serving:
Calories (kcal) 584.6
Protein (g) 53.6
Carbohydrates (g) 52.9
Total Sugars (g) 3.4
Dietary Fibre (g) 4.6
Fat (g) 18.7
Saturated Fat (g) 2.8

36% carbohydrate, GL:

6 Heat a griddle pan or grill and cook the salmon over high heat for 2-3 minutes each side, until seared on the outside but still a little underdone in the middle. Serve on a bed of noodles with the wasabi and pickled ginger on each piece of salmon.

Note: Buckwheat, the main component of soba noodles, has an amazing nutritional profile. It contains about 12-15% protein, including the essential amino acid lysine which is lacking in most cereal grains, and the flavonoids rutin and quercetin, both of which protect cholesterol in the blood from oxidation; high levels of magnesium – an important mineral for diabetics; high-quality protein; and chiro-inositol, which appears to prompt cells to become more insulin-sensitive. It's therefore one of the top ten anti-diabetic foods.

curried hoki with pineapple

Serves 4 Time taken: 30 minutes

4 Hoki fillets, about 170g/6 oz each
1 tbsp Coconut oil
1 Onion, peeled and finely chopped
2-3cm/1^1/$_2$" piece Fresh ginger root, peeled and grated
1 Lemongrass stalk, sliced
2 Kaffir lime leaves, sliced
3 tbsp Thai red curry paste
^{1}/$_2$ Fresh pineapple, peeled, cored and cubed (about 450g/1lb)
750ml/1^1/$_4$ pints (2^2/$_3$ cups) Coconut milk
12-15 Basil leaves
Small handful fresh coriander, leaves stripped off the stalks and torn roughly

1 Cut the fish into bite-sized pieces and set aside. Heat the coconut oil in a large saucepan and sauté the onion, ginger, lemongrass and kaffir lime leaves, stirring, until the onion is soft. Stir in the curry paste and cook for another few minutes. Add the fish pieces and toss gently for a minute or two, then add the pineapple. Pour in the coconut milk and cook over gentle heat for about 15-20 minutes, until the fish is cooked through.

2 Just before serving, stir in the basil leaves and torn coriander leaves. Serve with brown rice.

Note: Pineapple is very useful for people with poor digestion as it contains an enzyme, bromelain, which helps to break down protein bonds in the stomach. Many diabetics suffer from gastroparesis – slow stomach-emptying. This means that efficient breakdown of proteins in the stomach is especially important.

15% carbohydrate, GL: Ⓛ ● ●

Pineapple is a high GI fruit, but it is perfectly acceptable to eat it with a protein food, as in this fish curry. Hoki is a sustainable fish from New Zealand with a moist, white flesh and few bones – an excellent alternative to cod or haddock.

Per Serving:
Calories (kcal) 554.6
Protein (g) 41.8
Carbohydrates (g) 22.2
Total Sugars (g) 9.9
Dietary Fibre (g) 3.8
Fat (g) 37
Saturated Fat (g) 30.7

alaskan salmon with lettuce and fennel

Farmed salmon should be avoided and organic salmon is wildly expensive, so Alaskan salmon, which is on the Marine Conservation Society's list of 'fish to eat', is a reasonable alternative. It tastes quite different from Atlantic salmon, with a fine strong flavour and a deep red colour. This is a lovely, fresh recipe for spring.

Serves 2 **Time taken:** 25 minutes

2 Little gem lettuces, organic if possible
1 Small bulb fennel, thinly sliced
15g/$^1/_2$ oz (1 tbsp) Organic unsalted butter
120ml/4 fl oz ($^1/_2$ cup) White wine
2 x 200g/7 oz Wild Alaskan salmon fillets, skinned
2 tbsp Crème fraîche
Squeeze of lemon juice
Fresh chopped parsley or chervil, to serve

1 Trim and wash the whole lettuces, then plunge into boiling water, reduce the heat and cook for 3-4 minutes. Drain.

2 Melt the butter in a large pan with a lid. I usually use a large sauté pan with straight sides for this. Sauté the fennel lightly in the butter, then lay the drained lettuce on top of it. Pour over the wine, season, then cover and simmer for 10 minutes.

3 Lay the salmon on top of the lettuce, cover again and simmer gently for a further 10 minutes, until the fish is cooked. Take the salmon out carefully, then remove the lettuce and fennel with a slotted spoon. Pile the vegetables onto two hot plates, and place the salmon on top. Stir the crème fraîche into the cooking juices left in the pan, turn up the heat and boil to reduce slightly. Add a squeeze of lemon juice and adjust the seasoning. Pour the sauce over the salmon and serve hot, sprinkled with freshly chopped parsley or chervil.

Note: Fennel has a long history of medicinal use in the Mediterranean region, having traditionally been used for digestive ailments. It is an excellent source of vitamin C, potassium and dietary fibre. I like it best raw and thinly sliced in salads, but it also lends itself to cooking, which brings out its sweet anise-like flavour.

Per Serving:
Calories (kcal) 537.9
Protein (g) 57.3
Carbohydrates (g) 11.7
Total Sugars (g) 1.9
Dietary Fibre (g) 4.2
Fat (g) 23.6
Saturated Fat (g) 8.7

9% carbohydrate, GL: L ● ●

aromatic five spice trout

Serves 4 Time taken: 15-20 minutes

4 small Rainbow or brown trout (about 450g/1lb each), cleaned
2 tbsp Cornflour or potato flour
1 tsp Sea salt
1 tsp Chinese five spice powder
3 tbsp Groundnut oil
1 tbsp Finely chopped garlic
2 tsp Finely chopped fresh root ginger
3 tbsp Finely chopped spring onions
1 Lemon, quartered
4 Fresh coriander sprigs

1 Blot the trout dry inside and out with kitchen paper. Combine the cornflour or potato flour with the salt and five spice powder. Dust the trout on the outside with this mixture. Heat a large frying pan over a high heat. Add 2 tablespoons of the oil and, when it is very hot, turn the heat down to medium and pan fry the trout for about 4 minutes each side, until brown and crispy. You may have to do this in two batches. When the fish is cooked, transfer to a warm platter.

2 Wipe out the frying pan and reheat with the remaining oil. Add the garlic, ginger and spring onions and stir-fry for 2 minutes. Pour this mixture over the trout and serve garnished with the lemon wedges and fresh coriander sprigs.

Note: Trout are not only sustainable but very nutritious. It is true that they contain less omega 3 fatty acids than salmon, however they are a good source of lean protein and an excellent source of potassium, a mineral needed to help regulate blood pressure and water balance.

This is a Ken Hom recipe; very easy and very quick. I cook a lot of trout because my husband is a trout fisherman, and have found that the simple ways of cooking it are the best. If you prefer, you can fillet the fish, or get the fishmonger to do it for you, and cook the fillets as described below. They will take a little less time than the whole fish.

Per Serving:
Calories (kcal) 503.2
Protein (g) 55.4
Carbohydrates (g) 6.7
Total Sugars (g) 0.4
Dietary Fibre (g) 0.5
Fat (g) 26.9
Saturated Fat (g) 6.4

5% carbohydrate, GL: L ● ●

grilled sea bass with coriander yoghurt sauce and puréed lemons

This is a lovely, lemony, creamy fish dish with Mediterranean flavours, suitable for a summer evening.

Serves 6 **Time taken:** 35 minutes

3 **Lemons**
3 tsp **Honey**
1 small bunch **Fresh coriander**
400g/14 oz (1$\frac{1}{2}$ cups) **Natural Greek yoghurt**
Sea salt and freshly ground black pepper
1 **Cucumber**
1 tbsp **Extra virgin olive oil**
6 fillets of **Sea bass, about 170g/6 oz each**

1 Cut 2 of the lemons into quarters, slice thinly, then put in a pan. Cover with water and cook over a medium heat until there is only a little liquid left. Purée in the blender, adding 2 teaspoons of honey and the juice of half of the third lemon. Set aside the purée and wash the blender.

2 Put three quarters of the coriander and the yoghurt into the blender and purée, adding the juice from the last half lemon, salt and the remaining teaspoon of honey. Set aside.

3 Cut the cucumber in half, slice very thinly and mix with the rest of the coriander and a drizzle of olive oil. Set aside.

4 Heat the olive oil in a non-stick pan over medium-high heat. Season the pieces of fish and place in the pan skin side down. Cook for 5 minutes, until the skin is crispy and golden. Turn and cook for a further 2-3 minutes until cooked through. Divide the coriander sauce between 6 plates, add the cucumber salad and a spoonful of lemon purée. Place the fish on top of the cucumber and serve.

Note: Use farmed sea bass for this dish, which is a sustainable fish. It counts as an oily fish, being a good source of omega 3 fatty acids. It is also an excellent source of protein, together with magnesium and vitamin B6 which help to digest the protein in the stomach.

Per Serving:
Calories (kcal) 275.9
Protein (g) 37
Carbohydrates (g) 19.3
Total Sugars (g) 7
Dietary Fibre (g) 5.5
Fat (g) 8.4
Saturated Fat (g) 2.7

26% carbohydrate, GL: L ● ●

mackerel in crispy oatmeal

Serves 4 **Time taken:** 45 minutes

4 large Mackerel, filleted
90g/3 oz (1 cup) Medium oatmeal
1/2 tsp Sea salt
1/2 tsp Freshly ground black pepper
2 tbsp Plain or gluten-free flour
1 Free-range egg, beaten
2 tbsp Coconut oil
1 Lemon
Chopped parsley to serve

1 Check the fillets for bones. If you find any, remove them with tweezers.

2 Combine the oatmeal with the salt and pepper and spread on a plate. Coat the fillets in flour, then dip into the beaten egg, and finally into the oatmeal. Chill in the fridge for 10-15 minutes to set the coating. This helps to prevent it falling off the fish when you cook it.

3 Heat the coconut oil in a frying pan over medium heat and cook the fillets skin side down for about five minutes, then turn over and cook the other side for about the same length of time. The oats should be crispy and brown and the fish tender inside. Serve with wedges of lemon and garnish with chopped parsley.

Note: Mackerel is one of the oily fish, rich in omega 3 fatty acids, and contains a huge amount of magnesium – together with the oats, this dish delivers 144mg of magnesium per serving. Magnesium is probably the most important mineral for diabetics because it helps to promote insulin production. Many people are chronically short of magnesium in the diet, and body stores are easily depleted by stress, alcohol and prescription drugs.

Herring in oatmeal is a classic Scottish dish, but mackerel works just as well. If you haven't got medium oatmeal, you could whizz jumbo oats in the food processor for a few seconds.

Per Serving:
Calories (kcal) 560.6
Protein (g) 39.7
Carbohydrates (g) 18.3
Total Sugars (g) 0.3
Dietary Fibre (g) 3.0
Fat (g) 35.7
Saturated Fat (g) 12.7

15% carbohydrate, GL: ◐◯◯

roast sea bream
with romesco sauce

Serves 6 **Time taken:** 1 hour 25 minutes

For the sauce: 4 medium-size Ripe tomatoes
4 Cloves garlic
100ml/3 fl oz (1/3 cup) Extra-virgin olive oil
45g/1 1/2 oz (1/3 cup) Blanched almonds
45g/1 1/2 oz (1/4 cup) Hazelnuts
2 small Dried red chillies
1 tsp Sea salt; more to taste
2-3 tbsp Red wine vinegar
For the fish: 900g/2lb fillets of Sea bream
4 tbsp Extra virgin olive oil
Lemon juice
Sea salt and freshly ground black pepper
Garnish: 6 stalks of Cherry tomatoes on the vine

1 First, make the sauce. Preheat the oven to 190°C/375°F/gas 5. Put the tomatoes and garlic in a roasting pan and drizzle with 1 tbsp olive oil. Roast until caramelized but not burnt – about 50 minutes. Leave to cool. While the tomatoes roast, toast almonds and hazelnuts separately in the oven until browned, about 5-6 minutes. To rub the skins off the hazelnuts, roll in a clean tea towel.

2 Soak the dried chillies in hot water until soft, about 15 minutes. Chop roughly.

3 Put the roasted nuts and soaked chopped chillies into the food processor. When the tomatoes are cool, pull off their skins and put the flesh and the roasted garlic into the food processor together with the salt. Start the processor, adding the rest of the olive oil in a thin, steady stream, as for making mayonnaise. Add the vinegar at the end and taste for seasoning. The texture should be coarse and creamy at the same time. If it is a little thick, add a little more vinegar. Cover and set aside.

4 When you are ready to cook the fish, turn the oven up to 200°C/400°F/gas 6. Brush the fish with olive oil. Heat a large frying pan and add the rest of the olive oil, and fry the fish lightly on all sides. Transfer to a roasting pan and cook in the preheated oven for 10-15 minutes until cooked through. Roast the cherry tomatoes for the last five minutes, just until they start to collapse. Remove from the oven.

5 Season fish with salt, pepper and a squeeze of lemon juice. Serve with the Romesco sauce at room temperature, and garnish with the cherry tomatoes.

8% carbohydrate, GL:

Sea bream is on the Marine Conservation Society's list of sustainable fish. Organically farmed sea bream is available from Graig Farm Organics (see Useful Addresses). It has a thick skin and white flesh with a fine texture, and stands up well to roasting. Romesco sauce is a divine sauce from the Catalan city of Tarragona, made from tomatoes, nuts, chillies, garlic and olive oil. It has many variations and many uses – it can be served with salads, grilled vegetables, meat, chicken or fish, and keeps in the refrigerator for at least a week.

Per Serving:
Calories (kcal) 503.3
Protein (g) 33.5
Carbohydrates (g) 10.3
Total Sugars (g) 4.7
Dietary Fibre (g) 3.2
Fat (g) 37
Saturated Fat (g) 5

herring with mustard sauce

Serves 4 Time taken: 10 minutes

For the sauce: 15g/$^1/_2$ oz (1 tbsp) Organic unsalted butter
4 Shallots, finely chopped
50ml/2 fl oz ($^1/_4$ cup) White wine vinegar
150ml/5 fl oz ($^2/_3$ cup) Dry white wine
200g/7 oz ($^3/_4$ cup) Greek yoghurt
1$^1/_2$ tbsp Dijon mustard
A squeeze of lemon juice
Sea salt and freshly ground black pepper
For the fish: 8 Herrings, cleaned and filleted
A little seasoned flour, either plain or gluten-free
2 tbsp Coconut oil
A squeeze of lemon
1 tbsp Finely chopped flat leaf parsley

1 Melt the butter in a small pan and gently sauté the shallots until soft but not browned. Add the vinegar, increase the heat and reduce the liquid to about 2 teaspoons. Add the wine and reduce by half, then add the yoghurt, mustard and lemon juice. Taste and season.

2 Wash the fish and pat dry. Season on both sides, roll in seasoned flour (I do this by putting both fish and flour in a large plastic bag and shaking it around). Heat the coconut oil in a roomy frying pan and fry the fish, flesh side down, for one minute, then turn over and fry the other side for a further minute. Squeeze lemon juice over.

3 Spoon the sauce over the fish and serve with a scattering of parsley.

Note: With vitamin D levels up to 30mcg per 100g, herrings are the richest known source of this nutrient. More and more research is indicating that this vitamin can help protect against Type 2 diabetes, and improve insulin sensitivity in those who already have diabetes. Researchers have found that low blood levels of vitamin D interfere with the proper function of insulin-producing cells.

Herring are one of the most nutritious of fish, and much underrated in these modern times, perhaps because they contain a lot of bones or perhaps because they used to be the food of the poor. I'm glad to say that they are on the list of fish species that are not yet endangered, so they can be eaten with a clear conscience. Getting the fishmonger to fillet them for you should take care of the bone problem, and they taste good too.

Per Serving:
Calories (kcal) 462.3
Protein (g) 35.8
Carbohydrates (g) 9.6
Total Sugars (g) 3.3
Dietary Fibre (g) 0.3
Fat (g) 27.9
Saturated Fat (g) 12.5

8% carbohydrate, GL: **L** ● ●

seared prawns with chickpeas and puy lentils

This recipe comes from the resolutely Irish Richard Corrigan, but its influences are Middle Eastern.

Serves 4 **Time taken:** 45 minutes

60g/2 oz ($^1/_3$ cup) Chickpeas, or use half a 400g can of chickpeas, drained
100g/3$^1/_2$ oz ($^1/_2$ cup) Puy lentils
1 tsp Cumin seeds
6 tbsp Extra virgin olive oil (for cooking)
1 Onion, peeled and very finely diced
2 Garlic cloves, peeled and very finely diced
120ml/4 fl oz ($^1/_2$ cup) Water
$^1/_2$ Lemon, juice only
16-20 Large raw prawns (about 675g/1$^1/_2$ lbs)

1 Soak the chickpeas overnight, then drain and rinse. Put in a pan with plenty of water, bring to the boil for 10 minutes. Skim, then turn down to a simmer and cook until tender – 1$^1/_2$-2 hours depending on the age of the chickpeas. Drain and set aside. If you are using canned chickpeas, skip this step.

2 Cook the Puy lentils in another pan until tender but still holding their shape (about half an hour). Drain and set aside.

3 Heat a small frying pan and roast the cumin seeds over medium heat until fragrant. Remove and pound them lightly. Return the pan to the heat with one tablespoon of olive oil, and fry the onion and garlic for a couple of minutes over medium heat. Add the water and pounded cumin seeds, turn down the heat and cook for 10-15 minutes.

4 Combine the chickpeas and lentils with the onions, 4 tablespoons of olive oil and lemon juice. Season to taste.

5 Heat the remaining tablespoon of oil and cook the prawns briefly over very high heat, stirring constantly. Add them to the pulses with any juices from the pan and serve warm.

Note: Prawns are a rich source of calcium, needed for healthy bones and the cardiovascular system. Although they contain cholesterol, numerous studies demonstrate that dietary cholesterol does not raise blood cholesterol.
Of more concern is that the prawns you eat come from sustainable stocks or are ethically farmed. The Environmental Justice Foundation advises consumers to only buy shrimp/prawns with recognised, credible, environmental, Fair Trade and organic labels. For more information see: www.ejfoundation.org

Per Serving:
Calories (kcal) 458.2
Protein (g) 36.1
Carbohydrates (g) 25.1
Total Sugars (g) 2.9
Dietary Fibre (g) 6.4
Fat (g) 23.3
Saturated Fat (g) 3.4

20% carbohydrate, GL:

fragrant and hot prawns with green tea

Serves 4 **Time taken:** 15 minutes

675g/1¹/₂ lbs Tiger prawns, shelled and de-veined
¹/₂ tsp Sea salt
1 tbsp Chinese wine or dry sherry
300ml/¹/₂ pt (1¹/₄ cups) Groundnut oil
1 tsp Fresh ginger, peeled and finely chopped
1 Garlic clove, peeled and finely chopped
1 tsp Chilli bean paste
1 tsp Salted chillies (available in Chinese supermarkets)
2 tbsp Dried green tea leaves, soaked in hot water and drained
3 tbsp Water
Dark soy sauce, to taste
2 Spring onions, finely chopped
¹/₂ Red pepper, finely chopped
1 tsp Sesame oil

Green tea is one of the most powerful antioxidants in the nutritional armoury. In many parts of China it is fried with prawns. It is hard to find sustainable sources of tiger prawns, so you could use farmed Dublin Bay prawns instead, which are sustainable but expensive.

1 Rinse the prawns and mix with the salt and wine or sherry and set aside. Heat the oil in a wok over high heat. Shake the prawns dry and deep fry them in the wok for less than 30 seconds, until they turn pink. Remove and set aside.

2 Discard all but 3 tbsp of the oil and return the wok to a medium heat. Add the ginger, garlic, chilli bean paste, chopped salted chillies and half the soaked green tea leaves, reserving the other half for a garnish. Stir fry until the oil is fragrant and deep red from the chillies. Add the water and a few drops of dark soy sauce and bring to the boil.

3 Add the prawns and cook for a minute or two over high heat, stirring constantly, until the sauce has more or less evaporated. Add the spring onions and red pepper, stir once, then take off the heat. Add the sesame oil and serve garnished with the reserved green tea leaves.

Note: The health benefits of green tea derive from its polyphenol content. Not only are these antioxidant, but they appear to increase the activity of antioxidant enzymes in the small intestine, liver and lungs. A number of studies have shown that they inhibit the formation of cancer-causing compounds. In addition to this, animal studies suggest that green tea may help prevent the development of Type 1 diabetes and slow the progression once it has developed.

Per Serving:
Calories (kcal) 343
Protein (g) 36.7
Carbohydrates (g) 9.4
Total Sugars (g) 1.3
Dietary Fibre (g) 0.8
Fat (g) 17.2
Saturated Fat (g) 2.3

11% carbohydrate, GL: L ● ●

beans and whole grains

tarka dahl

Serves 4 Time taken: 1 hour

170g/6 oz (^{3}/$_4$ cup) Red lentils (masoor dahl)
600ml/1 pt (2^2/$_3$ cups) Water
1 tsp Ground turmeric
1 tsp Ground cumin
Sea salt to taste
2 tbsp Groundnut oil
1 medium Onion, peeled and finely chopped
2.5cm/1" piece Ginger root, peeled and grated
2 Garlic cloves, peeled and finely chopped
2 Dried red chillies, chopped
1 tsp Cumin seeds

1 Combine dahl, water, turmeric, cumin and salt in a saucepan, and bring mixture to a boil. Turn heat down to medium and cook, uncovered, for 8-10 minutes, stirring often.

2 Cover the pan, turn down the heat and simmer for 30 minutes, stirring occasionally. Remove from heat and let cool slightly. At this point, you can purée the mixture in a food processor or blender if you like it really smooth, but it is not necessary to do this.

3 For the 'tarka', heat the groundnut oil in a small pan over medium heat. Fry the onion, ginger, garlic and red chillies until the onions are browned (8-10 minutes). Stir in the cumin seeds for the last couple of minutes. Stir half of the onion mixture into the dahl. Transfer to a serving dish and garnish with the rest of the onion mixture.

Note: Red lentils are rich in minerals, especially magnesium, iron, zinc and calcium. Of the pulse family, they are second only to soybeans in protein value, and contain a good amount of fibre.

Dahl means both lentils and any dish made with lentils. There are probably as many recipes for dahl as there are cooks in India. This is a very basic dahl, which goes with any Indian meal, and makes a complete protein if eaten with brown rice.

Per Serving:
Calories (kcal) 158.8
Protein (g) 7.6
Carbohydrates (g) 17.9
Total Sugars (g) 1.7
Dietary Fibre (g) 6.9
Fat (g) 7
Saturated Fat (g) 4.1

43% carbohydrate, GL: ● Ⓜ ●

spiced red beans in coconut milk

Beans in coconut milk are eaten all over East Africa. This version, called Maharagwe, is from Kenya.

Serves 4 **Time taken:** 2 hours plus soaking

200g/7 oz (1 cup) **Dried red kidney beans, soaked overnight**
2 medium **Onions, peeled and chopped**
1-2 tbsp **Coconut oil**
2-3 **Tomatoes, peeled and chopped**
1 tsp **Sea salt**
2 tsp **Turmeric**
3 **Dried chillies, ground to a paste, or use** 1 1/2 **tsp cayenne pepper**
450ml/16 fl oz (2 cups) **Coconut milk**

1 Drain the beans of their soaking water and place in a large pot with fresh, cold water to cover. Bring to the boil, reduce the heat, cover and simmer until they are just tender. Timing depends on the freshness of the beans – older ones will take longer – but should be about 1 1/2 hours. By this time most of the water should have reduced to a thick liquid. If not, boil hard for a few minutes to reduce.

2 Heat the coconut oil in a frying pan over medium heat and sauté the onions until golden. Add to the beans, together with the rest of the ingredients. Simmer for another 15-20 minutes or so until the beans are tender and the tomatoes are cooked. Taste for seasoning and serve very hot with a wholegrain such as brown rice or buckwheat.

Note: This dish contains more dietary fibre than any other recipe in this book. Fibre, whilst having very little nutritional value, is very important for the health of the digestive system. If you are not used to eating so much fibre, it might be wise to try a small portion first. Beans can cause flatulence in people whose digestive system is not used to them, but cooking the beans with a piece of root ginger or a piece of kombu seaweed can help to break down the carbohydrates that cause flatulence.

Per Serving:
Calories (kcal) 425.8
Protein (g) 13
Carbohydrates (g) 31.7
Total Sugars (g) 1.9
Dietary Fibre (g) 12.3
Fat (g) 30.1
Saturated Fat (g) 26.3

28% carbohydrate, GL: M

fassolada

Serves 6 **Time taken:** 2 hours plus soaking

300g/10 1/2 oz (1 3/4 cup) Haricot beans or butterbeans, soaked overnight
2 tbsp Extra virgin olive oil
3 Carrots, peeled unless organic, and sliced thickly
4 Celery sticks, sliced
3 tbsp Celery leaves, chopped
1 large Onion, finely sliced
3 large Ripe tomatoes, skinned and chopped
Sea salt and freshly ground black pepper
To serve: 6 Lemon wedges
2 tbsp Extra virgin olive oil

1 Drain the beans, rinse well and put in a large pan with cold water to cover. Bring to the boil, boil hard for 5 minutes, then drain again and throw the water away. (This is the way my Greek hostess dealt with the unfortunate digestive effect beans can sometimes produce.)

2 Add the onion, carrots, celery and the chopped leaves, and olive oil. Cover with water. Bring to a simmer and cook for about 1 1/2 hours, adding more water if necessary.

3 After an hour, add the chopped tomatoes and seasoning. Continue cooking until the beans are tender and the liquid has reduced to a thick sauce.

4 Adjust the seasoning and serve piping hot in wide shallow bowls with a wedge of lemon and an extra drizzle of olive oil.

Note: Haricot beans are a particularly good source of soluble fibre, which has been found to reduce blood cholesterol levels. They also contain more calcium and magnesium than any of the other pulses except soybeans.

This dish could belong in the soup chapter as well as here. It is a wonderfully comforting soup/stew from Greece, where I spent one winter in the 1970s as the guest of a family in Athens. Fassolada is typical of the food I ate there at that time of the year. This makes a large quantity, but you will easily eat it all – it tastes even better the second day.

Per Serving:
Calories (kcal) 296.5
Protein (g) 13.2
Carbohydrates (g) 40.9
Total Sugars (g) 6
Dietary Fibre (g) 10.5
Fat (g) 10.1
Saturated Fat (g) 1.5

53% carbohydrate, GL: ● Ⓜ ●

chana dahl with coconut and whole spices

This delicious Bengali dish is adapted from David Mendosa's comprehensive list of chana dahl recipes. It is quite sweet, due to the raisins and coconut, but not cloying. Don't be put off by the long list of ingredients; it's really worth using whole spices here instead of a curry powder. You can buy chana dahl in Asian shops and some supermarkets. It has the lowest GI (11) and GL (4) of any pulse – hence its popularity with diabetics.

Serves 4 **Time taken:** 1¹/₂ hours plus soaking

285g/10 oz (1¹/₂ cups) Chana dahl (Bengal gram), washed, then soaked overnight
1 tsp Turmeric
2.5cm/1" piece Root ginger, peeled
1 whole Fresh green chilli
¹/₂ tsp Sea salt
3 tsp Ground cumin
3 tbsp Raisins
2 tbsp Coconut oil
1 Bay leaf, crumbled
1 whole Dried red chilli
6 Cardamom pods
1 Cinnamon stick
4 whole Cloves
¹/₂ tsp Black mustard seeds
1 tbsp Chopped fresh green chilli (or to taste)
3 tbsp Desiccated coconut
1 tsp Garam masala
Lemon wedges and whole coriander leaves, to serve

1 Drain the chana dahl. Put it in a large pan with 1.5 litres/2³/₄ pints water. Bring to the boil over medium heat. Add the turmeric, ginger and whole green chilli. Simmer, covered, for an hour or until the dahl is very tender and breaks easily when pressed between thumb and index finger. Stir the dahl often, adding 1 to 2 tablespoons of hot water if it starts to stick to the bottom. Discard the whole chilli and ginger. Add salt and cumin and remove from the heat.

2 Purée a cupful (about 170g/6 oz) of the dahl mixture in a blender, adding a little water if necessary. Return to the pan and add the raisins. Bring to a simmer, then keep warm.

3 Heat the coconut oil in a small pan over medium low heat. Add the bay leaf and red chilli and cook until the chilli darkens. Add the cardamom, cinnamon, and cloves and fry for 5 seconds. Add the black mustard seeds and fry for another few seconds. Turn the heat to low, add the chopped green chilli and coconut and cook for a few seconds, stirring constantly. Remove from the heat. Add this spice mixture to the dahl and simmer for 2 to 3 more minutes. Remove from the heat and stir in the garam masala. Garnish with lemon wedges, sprinkle with whole coriander leaves, and serve hot.

43% carbohydrate, GL:

Per Serving:
Calories (kcal) 303.5
Protein (g) 8.5
Carbohydrates (g) 34.2
Total Sugars (g) 10.6
Dietary Fibre (g) 10.3
Fat (g) 16.4
Saturated Fat (g) 12.2

sambhar

Serves 6 **Time taken:** 15 minutes

225g/8 oz (³/₄ cup) **Red (masoor dahl) or yellow lentils (toor dahl)**
2 tbsp **Coriander seeds**
10 **Black peppercorns**
¹/₂ tsp **Fenugreek seeds**
2 tbsp **Grated fresh coconut or desiccated coconut**
1 tbsp **Roasted chana dahl (Bengal gram)**
6 **Dried red chillies**
450g/1 lb **mixed vegetables (such as cauliflower, courgettes, red peppers, okra,**
   mushrooms, peas, Brussels sprouts), chopped
1 tbsp **Tamarind purée**
2 tbsp **Coconut oil**
1 tsp **Black mustard seeds**
10 **Curry leaves**
¹/₂ tsp **Ground turmeric**
¹/₂ tsp **Asafoetida**
Sea salt to taste

1 Pick over the lentils, wash them and put in a saucepan with 1 litre/1³/₄ pts/4 cups water. Bring to the boil, then reduce the heat, cover and simmer until tender, 30-40 minutes.

2 While the lentils are cooking, dry roast the coriander, peppercorns, fenugreek, coconut, chana dahl and chillies, stirring constantly until the coconut is golden brown. Fenugreek seeds burn very easily so watch the mixture carefully. Cool a little, then grind in a spice grinder or with a pestle and mortar.

3 Now, cook the vegetables. Put a large pan of water to boil, and steam them until barely tender – not more than 5 minutes.

4 Put the cooked lentils and any remaining liquid, the ground spices, vegetables and tamarind purée in a large saucepan and simmer for 20 minutes or so, until all the flavours are amalgamated. You may have to add a little water.

5 Heat the oil in a small saucepan over medium heat, add the mustard seeds, cover and shake the pan until they start to pop. Add the curry leaves, turmeric, asafoetida and salt to taste. Pour over the dahl and stir to mix. Serve with quick soya dhosas (see page 57) or with brown rice.

Note: In India chana dahl is sold ready roasted. When roasted it puffs up and has a crunchy texture. You can roast your own in a dry pan with a lid.

49% carbohydrate, GL:

Sambhar is a savoury South Indian mixture of lentils and vegetables, a favourite Indian breakfast accompaniment to idli (rice dumplings) or dhosas (pancakes). The recipe looks long but it's not difficult.

Per Serving:
Calories (kcal) 242.2
Protein (g) 12.3
Carbohydrates (g) 31.9
Total Sugars (g) 5
Dietary Fibre (g) 12.7
Fat (g) 9.2
Saturated Fat (g) 6.8

Black turtle beans are a small variety of black haricot beans, worth seeking out as they have a rich taste and keep their shape well when cooked. They are not the same as Asian black beans, which are a type of fermented soya bean. These spicy bean cakes are typical of Caribbean and Central American cuisine and would traditionally be fried, but I bake them to reduce the fat. The onion marmalade is made without sugar but caramalises with long, slow cooking.

Per Serving:
Calories (kcal) 305.5
Protein (g) 13.4
Carbohydrates (g) 32.6
Total Sugars (g) 4.2
Dietary Fibre (g) 10.6
Fat (g) 14.5
Saturated Fat (g) 2.1

black bean cakes with ginger onion marmalade

Serves 6 **Time taken:** 2 hours plus soaking

225g/8 oz (1¼ cups) Black turtle beans, soaked overnight
2.5cm/1" piece Root ginger, peeled
1 tbsp Extra virgin olive oil
1 Medium onion, finely chopped
2 Organic free-range eggs
60g/2 oz (½ cup) Ground almonds
2 Garlic cloves, finely chopped
1 Stick celery, thinly sliced
2 tsp Ground cumin
1 tsp Ground allspice
Pinch of cayenne pepper, or to taste
Sea salt and freshly ground black pepper
For the onion marmalade: 450g/1lb Onions, peeled and sliced as thinly as possible
2 tbsp Extra virgin olive oil
1 tbsp Freshly grated ginger
Sea salt to taste

1 Drain the beans of their soaking water, cover with fresh water and add the ginger. Bring to the boil, then simmer steadily for about 1½ hours until the beans are tender. Drain, discard the piece of ginger and leave the beans to cool.

2 Meanwhile, for the onion marmalade, heat the oil over medium heat in a wok or large frying pan. Add the onions, stirring and breaking the slices into rings as you go. Cover the pan with a lid, and leave the onions to sweat over a very low heat for 30 minutes. Remove the lid, add the salt and grated ginger, and stir fry the onions for another 10 minutes uncovered to remove any excess moisture. The onions should be soft and melting. Set aside for the flavours to mingle while you prepare the bean cakes.

3 Mash the beans coarsely with a potato masher until they start sticking together. Alternatively you could purée them in the processor, but if you do this only purée about a quarter of the beans and leave the rest whole, to give some texture. Put the mashed beans in a large bowl and add the beaten eggs and ground almonds.

4 Heat the olive oil in a pan over medium heat. Add the onion, garlic and celery and sauté until very tender and beginning to brown, about 10 minutes. Stir in the cumin, allspice and cayenne, and cook for another minute or two.

42% carbohydrate, GL:

5 Stir the sautéed vegetables into the bean mixture and season to taste. Stir to mix well.

6 Preheat the oven to 190°C/375°F/Gas Mark 5. Lightly oil a baking sheet. Using your hands, form the bean mixture into 12 round cakes, flattening them with a palette knife, and place on the baking sheet. Bake in the preheated oven for 10 minutes, then take them out, turn them over and bake for 10 more minutes. Serve the bean cakes with the onion marmalade on the side.

Note: All of this dish, except the final baking, can be prepared in advance. Serve the bean cakes and onion marmalade with a large green salad.

quinoa with herbs and pomegranate

Serves 4 **Time taken:** 25 minutes

200g/7 oz (1 cup) Quinoa
175ml/6 fl oz (³/4 cup) Water or vegetable stock
2 tbsp Extra virgin olive oil
Sea salt and freshly ground black pepper
2 Pomegranates
30g/1 oz (2 tbsp) Shelled, unsalted pistachio nuts, chopped
Squeeze of lemon juice
3 tbsp Flat leaf parsley, roughly chopped
3 tbsp Mint leaves, roughly chopped

1 Wash the quinoa well, then cook in water or stock over a low heat until tender but just holding its shape (about 20 minutes), by which time the liquid should have evaporated. Stir in the olive oil and seasoning.

2 Meanwhile, halve the pomegranates, and extract the seeds with a teaspoon, discarding the bitter white membrane. Stir into the quinoa together with the pistachios, lemon juice and herbs. Serve warm.

Note: Pomegranates are a 'superfood' as they have exceptionally high levels of polyphenols – antioxidants that prevent free radical damage by limiting the build-up of plaque in the arteries. Eating pomegranates can lower blood pressure and may even slow down the ageing process. As for quinoa, it was one of the most sacred foods of the Incas, a plant so nourishing, delicious and vital, they called it chesiya mama; the 'mother grain'. Apart from its excellent amino acid profile, it is one of the very best sources of magnesium, an important mineral for diabetics. A portion of this pilaf provides 129mg of magnesium.

68% carbohydrate, GL:

This was originally a couscous recipe from the Middle East, but to lighten the 'wheat load' I use the versatile quinoa instead of couscous. The result is a sweet and nutty pilaff that can be eaten on its own or as an accompaniment to meat dishes.

Per Serving:
Calories (kcal) 295.3
Protein (g) 9.4
Carbohydrates (g) 53.0
Total Sugars (g) 13.6
Dietary Fibre (g) 5.4
Fat (g) 6.6
Saturated Fat (g) 0.8

sweet cinnamon rice

Many cuisines of the world use rice as a staple. This dish features cinnamon, known to help reduce blood sugar levels, and I have substituted brown rice for the more usual white rice, because it has a lower GI.

Serves 6 **Time taken:** 50 minutes

45g/1^1/$_2$ oz (3 tbsp) Organic unsalted butter
1 Onion, peeled and finely chopped
2 sticks Celery, finely chopped
^{3}/$_4$ tbsp Ground cinnamon
30g/1 oz (2 tbsp) Raisins
340g/12 oz (1^3/$_4$ cups) Brown basmati rice
Sea salt and freshly ground black pepper
1 litre/1^3/$_4$ pints (4 cups) Boiling water or stock
2 tbsp Fresh coriander leaves, roughly chopped

1 Melt the butter in a heavy bottomed pan and cook the onion and celery until soft and golden. Add the cinnamon and cook for a minute, then add the raisins and the rice. Stir until the rice is coated in butter, season to taste, then add the water or stock. Bring to the boil, reduce the heat to a gentle simmer, cover and cook for 30-35 minutes without stirring, until all the liquid is absorbed and the rice is cooked. Leave to steam for a further five minutes, then fork through and add the coriander. Serve as a side dish with meat or chicken.

Note: Cinnamon rice is a natural partner for curries and dahls, but it is wise for diabetics to keep the proportion of rice to curry low to moderate the effect on blood sugar, so serve half as much rice as curry.

Per Serving:
Calories (kcal) 281.9
Protein (g) 4.3
Carbohydrates (g) 51.3
Total Sugars (g) 4.7
Dietary Fibre (g) 3.3
Fat (g) 7.3
Saturated Fat (g) 3.8

71% carbohydrate, GL: ● ● **H**

brown basmati biryani

Serves 4 Time taken: 1^1/$_2$ hours

225g/8 oz (1 cup) Brown basmati rice
2 tbsp Coconut oil
4 Garlic cloves, crushed
4cm/2" Piece of root ginger, peeled and grated
4 Medium onions, peeled and finely chopped
6 Whole cardamom pods
3 Whole cloves
^{1}/$_2$ tsp Sea salt
1 tsp Ground turmeric
4 Tomatoes, peeled and chopped
60g/2 oz Paneer (see page 142)
110g/4 oz (1^1/$_2$ cups) Grated fresh or frozen coconut
8-10 Mild green chillies, deseeded and sliced lengthwise
12 Green beans, topped, tailed and cut in half
^{1}/$_2$ Cauliflower, cut into small florets
1 handful Mint leaves, chopped
1 handful Coriander leaves, chopped
2 tsp Ground cinnamon
1 Lime, cut into quarters

1 First, cook the rice. Soak it for 20 minutes in cold water. Then rinse and put in a pan with a pinch of salt and cover with water to 1cm/ 1/1/2" above the surface of the rice. Bring to the boil and cook uncovered for 15 minutes. Cover the pan, turn down the heat and simmer for five minutes more. Turn off the heat and leave to steam for a further five minutes. Take off the lid and fork through the rice. Allow to cool.

2 Heat the coconut oil over medium heat, then add the garlic, ginger and onions. Sauté, stirring, until golden brown. Add the cardamoms, cloves, salt and turmeric, and then the chopped tomatoes. Add the paneer, coconut and chillies, and cook for 10 minutes.

3 Meanwhile, steam the beans and cauliflower separately over boiling water until just tender.

4 Add the rice to the onion mixture, together with a tablespoon each of chopped mint and chopped coriander, then stir in the cooked vegetables. Pack into an ovenproof casserole and keep warm in a low oven for about half an hour.

5 Serve garnished with the remaining mint and coriander, a sprinkle of cinnamon and a wedge of lime.

53% carbohydrate, GL: ● ● Ⓗ

Brown rice is not much used in Indian cooking, but as it is so much more nutritious than white rice, it is worth searching out brown basmati rice, the king of Indian rice varieties. This biryani is a version of the classic Punjabi dish.

Note: The sprinkling of cinnamon should not be overlooked, as it is an effective blood-sugar lowering agent.

Per Serving:
Calories (kcal) 415.6
Protein (g) 8.6
Carbohydrates (g) 58.1
Total Sugars (g) 6.3
Dietary Fibre (g) 7.6
Fat (g) 19.1
Saturated Fat (g) 15.3

seven vegetable kasha with apricots

This is an adaptation of a Moroccan couscous dish. Most couscous is made from refined wheat or millet, both of which are high GI, so I have substituted roasted buckwheat, also known as kasha, which makes this hearty dish suitable for celiacs since buckwheat is a non-gluten grain. Buckwheat can be rather dry, so serving it with a sauce in this way works very well.

Serves 6 Time taken: 45 minutes

170g/6 oz (1 cup) Roasted buckwheat groats (kasha)
530ml/18 fl oz (2 1/4 cups) Boiling water
2 tbsp Extra virgin olive oil
2 medium Onions, peeled and quartered
2 medium Carrots, cut into chunks
1 400g/14 oz can Chickpeas, drained and rinsed
110g/4 oz (1 cup) Cashew nuts
2 large Courgettes, cut into chunks
2 Red peppers cut into 5cm/2" squares
450g/1lb Sweet potatoes, peeled and cut into small chunks
2 large Tomatoes, sliced
100g/3 1/2 oz (1/2 cup) Dried apricots, halved
1 tsp Turmeric
Cayenne pepper
1 stick Cinnamon
4 Whole cloves
1 Bay leaf
Sea salt and freshly ground black pepper
To serve: Harissa (see page 147)

1 Wash the kasha well and put into a saucepan, pour in the boiling water. Turn down the heat to a very gentle simmer, cover the pan tightly and simmer for 30 minutes without stirring. Remove from the heat and leave for 5 minutes.

2 Meanwhile, cook the vegetables. Heat the olive oil in a large pan over medium heat and cook the onions and carrots for 5 minutes or so, until starting to brown and soften. Then add all the other ingredients. Stir the mixture, then add enough water to cover. Bring to the boil and simmer gently for 20-30 minutes, or until the vegetables are tender.

3 Put the kasha on a large serving plate, then remove the vegetables from their cooking liquid using a slotted spoon, and arrange on top of the kasha. Keep warm. Boil up the sauce and cook hard to reduce to about 300ml/1/2 pt/1 1/4 cups. Serve the sauce in a jug, and also serve harissa for those who like their food hot and spicy.

P er Serving:
Calories (kcal) 405.4
Protein (g) 12.6
Carbohydrates (g) 59.6
Total Sugars (g) 12.9
Dietary Fibre (g) 11.1
Fat (g) 15.5
Saturated Fat (g) 2.4

56% carbohydrate, GL:

salads and vegetables

thai cabbage salad with lime and coconut dressing

This is a wonderful way to perk up a white or green cabbage. The very quick cooking just softens the cabbage slightly and takes the raw edge off.

Serves 6 **Time taken:** 15 minutes

3 large Fresh red chillies
2 tbsp Ground nut oil
6 Garlic cloves, peeled and sliced
6 Shallots, peeled and sliced
1/2 Green or white cabbage, finely shredded
1 tbsp Peanuts, roughly chopped or crushed
For the dressing: 2 tbsp Thai fish sauce (Nam Pla)
2 tbsp Fresh lime juice
120ml/4 fl oz (1/2 cup) Coconut milk

1 Cut the chillies into thin strips and discard the seeds. Heat the oil in a wok or frying pan over medium heat, and stir fry the chillies until lightly browned and crisp. Remove and drain on kitchen paper, and repeat with the garlic and then the shallots.

2 Plunge the shredded cabbage into a large pan of boiling water, leave it in the water for 30 seconds only, then drain immediately.

3 For the dressing, mix all the ingredients together in a bowl.

4 Combine the cabbage with the dressing and toss well. Serve the salad topped with the stir-fried chillies, garlic and shallots, and sprinkled with chopped peanuts.

Note: Cabbage has something of an image problem, even though we all know that it is good for us. That's why attractive ways of incorporating it into the diet, such as this salad, are so valuable. Cabbage is a good source of vitamin K which protects the body from insulin resistance. Cabbage leaves have anti-inflammatory effects, both inside and outside the body. Choose the dark outer leaves as they contain 50 times more carotene than the pale inner leaves.

Per Serving:
Calories (kcal) 137.1
Protein (g) 3.2
Carbohydrates (g) 11.3
Total Sugars (g) 1.8
Dietary Fibre (g) 0.8
Fat (g) 10.2
Saturated Fat (g) 4.5

30% carbohydrate, GL: (L)●●

egyptian broad bean salad

Serves 4 Time taken: 20 minutes

1.8kg/4 lbs Fresh broad beans in the pod
Fresh sage leaves
4 Organic free range eggs, hard boiled
1 tbsp Fresh coriander leaves

For the dressing:
3 tbsp Extra virgin olive oil
1 tbsp Fresh lemon juice
2 tsp Dried red chilli pepper flakes
1 tbsp Whole cumin seeds, dry roasted
Sea salt and freshly ground black pepper

1 Shell the broad beans – you should have about 675g/1^1/$_2$ lbs of beans after shelling – and cook in boiling water for 10 minutes with a few sage leaves. Drain and plunge into cold water until cool enough to handle, then slip off the outer skins. (If the beans are very young and tender you can skip this step.) Shell the eggs and cut them into quarters.

2 Mix together all the ingredients for the dressing. Pour over the beans and toss very gently to mix. Arrange on a serving platter surrounded by the egg quarters and garnish with coriander leaves.

Note: Broad beans are good sources of protein, fibre, vitamins A and C, potassium and iron. They also contain levodopa (L-dopa), a chemical the body uses to produce dopamine (the neurotransmitter associated with the brain's reward and motivation system), so in theory they should make you feel calm and contented.

There is a wonderful Egyptian dish made with dried brown broad beans called ful medames. This is a variation made with fresh broad beans, best made with the first beans of the season before they have grown their thick skins, as it is a bit tedious to remove them, though well worth the trouble.

Per Serving:
Calories (kcal) 209
Protein (g) 8.5
Carbohydrates (g) 18.6
Total Sugars (g) 0.2
Dietary Fibre (g) 6.5
Fat (g) 11.8
Saturated Fat (g) 1.8

35% carbohydrate, GL: L ● ●

This is a very simple side salad, and makes a refreshing change from the ubiquitous green leaf salad. I like it made with tart green apples such as Granny Smiths.

greek apple salad

Serves 4 Time taken: 10 minutes

3 Green apples, cored and chopped but not peeled
1 large Mild Spanish onion, peeled and cut into rings
4 tbsp Plain live yoghurt (see page 140)
Pinch of freshly ground black pepper
1 Lemon, juice only
60g/2 oz (4 tbsp) Feta cheese, crumbled
1 tbsp Chopped fresh flat-leaf parsley

1 Simply combine the apples, onion, yoghurt, black pepper and lemon juice. Sprinkle with crumbled feta cheese and serve garnished with chopped parsley.

Note: The pectin in apples can help to keep blood sugar levels stable. The natural sugars in apples are digested and absorbed slowly. This is probably partly due to the effect of the pectin, which forms a gel in the digestive tract. The slow rise in blood sugar levels caused by apples means that they have a low GI, which makes them particularly useful for people with diabetes.

Per Serving:
Calories (kcal) 108.6
Protein (g) 3.9
Carbohydrates (g) 19.2
Total Sugars (g) 12.7
Dietary Fibre (g) 3.2
Fat (g) 2.6
Saturated Fat (g) 1.7

66% carbohydrate, GL: ● Ⓜ ●

indian stir-fry salad

Serves 4 **Time taken:** 15 minutes

1 tsp Groundnut oil
1 tsp Onion seeds
1 Green pepper, cut into thin strips
1 Spring onion, sliced
110g/4 oz (1/2 cup) Baby corn, sliced
1/2 Cucumber, sliced
110g/4 oz (1/2 cup) Broccoli florets
60g/2 oz (1/4 cup) Bean sprouts
1 small Tomato, deseeded and sliced
Sea salt to taste
110g/4 oz (1 cup) Paneer, cut into thin strips (see page 142)

1 Heat the oil in a wok or large sauté pan and add the onion seeds. Add all the vegetables and salt and stir-fry over high heat till the vegetables are tender.

2 Add the paneer and sauté for another minute. Remove from the heat and serve immediately.

Note: You could substitute strips of tofu for the paneer, as they don't really need any cooking. Tofu would considerably raise the protein content of this dish.

A colourful assortment of vegetables tossed lightly with paneer and onion seeds, this is a hot salad.

Per Serving:
Calories (kcal) 98.5
Protein (g) 5.4
Carbohydrates (g) 17.9
Total Sugars (g) 3.2
Dietary Fibre (g) 3.3
Fat (g) 1.9
Saturated Fat (g) 0.3

65% carbohydrate, GL: ● M ●

japanese tuna, watercress and radish salad

This is an elegant salad which you could serve in small portions as a starter, or for a light meal in itself. It's high in protein and very low GL.

Serves 4 Time taken: 15 minutes

450g/1 lb Tuna loin
1 scant tsp Freshly ground black pepper
1 tbsp Coconut oil
1 tbsp Rice wine vinegar
2 handfuls Watercress
12 Radishes, very finely sliced
1/2 small Red onion, very finely sliced into rings
For the dressing: 1/2 tbsp Wholegrain mustard
2 tsp Freshly grated ginger
1 tbsp Tamari sauce
1 tbsp Rice vinegar
4 tbsp Extra virgin olive oil

1 Sprinkle the tuna all over with pepper. Heat the coconut oil in a frying pan until hot. Add the tuna and cook briefly on all sides. If you prefer your tuna 'seared' rather than cooked, cook only until the tuna turns white, otherwise cook for about 5 minutes in total. Set aside and pour the rice wine vinegar over it.

2 For the dressing, mix everything together with a fork.

3 Cut the tuna into very thin slices, using a sharp knife. Place on four plates. Toss the watercress, radishes and onions together and arrange in a pile beside the tuna. Drizzle the dressing over the salad and the fish and serve.

Note: Tuna is a magnificent source of omega 2 fatty acids and protein. However, some species are endangered and fishing methods questionable. Choose line-caught or troll-caught 'dolphin friendly' tuna where possible. Albacore, skipjack and yellowfin are all good choices as they are currently being fished at sustainable levels.

Per Serving:
Calories (kcal) 383
Protein (g) 34.9
Carbohydrates (g) 4
Total Sugars (g) 1.2
Dietary Fibre (g) 0.4
Fat (g) 24.6
Saturated Fat (g) 6.7

4% carbohydrate, GL: ●●●

thai salad of prawns and grapefruit

Serves 4 **Time taken:** 5 minutes

$1/2$ **large Red chilli, deseeded**
Pinch of salt
4 tbsp Lime juice
3 tbsp Thai fish sauce
225g/8 oz ($1/2$ pound) Blanched, peeled prawns
2 Pink grapefruit, peeled and segmented
2 stalks Lemongrass, finely sliced
2 Shallots, sliced
2-3 tbsp Toasted, shredded coconut, preferably fresh or frozen

1 Chop the chilli very finely and mix with the salt, lime juice and fish sauce. This can be done with a pestle and mortar. Combine with the remaining ingredients and serve.

Note: Grapefruit, which has a very low GI, may be one of the healthiest dietary choices for people with diabetes and for those trying to lose weight, because it contains enzymes that help control insulin spikes that occur after a meal, thus freeing the digestive system to process food more efficiently, with the result that fewer nutrients are stored as fat.

This salad has a lovely fresh taste and, apart from segmenting the grapefruit, is very quick to make and needs no cooking. At a pinch, you could use grapefruit canned in its own juice.

Per Serving:
Calories (kcal) 169.6
Protein (g) 14.6
Carbohydrates (g) 21.1
Total Sugars (g) 12.4
Dietary Fibre (g) 2.7
Fat (g) 4.3
Saturated Fat (g) 3

46% carbohydrate, GL: **M**

vietnamese table salad

I've never been to Vietnam but have often enjoyed eating in Vietnamese restaurants. A table salad is often part of the meal. Having a plate of raw vegetables, salad leaves and fresh herbs on the table is an excellent habit to adopt at home. The sauce is a variation of the traditional dipping sauce. I have reduced the sugar but not eliminated it completely otherwise the sauce would be very sour.

Serves 6 **Time taken:** 10 minutes

1 Lettuce, either cos or iceberg
$1/2$ **Cucumber, peeled and thinly sliced**
1-2 Carrots, peeled and thinly sliced
225g/8 oz (2 cups) Mung bean sprouts
Small bunch of coriander, stalks removed
Small bunch of Thai basil or ordinary basil, stalks removed
Small bunch of mint, stalks removed
For the sauce: **1 small Hot red chilli, deseeded and roughly chopped**
1 Garlic clove, peeled and roughly chopped
1 tbsp Brown sugar
60ml/2 fl oz ($1/4$ cup) Warm water
2 tbsp Fresh lime juice
60ml/2 fl oz ($1/4$ cup) Rice vinegar
60ml/2 fl oz ($1/4$ cup) Vietnamese fish sauce (nuoc mam)

1 Separate the lettuce leaves, wash and dry. Arrange in a pile on a large plate. Arrange the sliced cucumber and carrots next to the lettuce, and the other ingredients in piles.

2 For the sauce, combine all the ingredients in a blender or food processor and process for 30 seconds, or until the sugar dissolves. Pour into a small serving bowl and serve with the salad. This sauce keeps for up to 2 weeks in the fridge, but is at its best when freshly made.

3 It's traditional to use a lettuce leaf to wrap a small parcel of salad and dip it in the sauce.

Note: **This salad takes minutes to make, and the ingredients can be varied according to what you have to hand. Try different kinds of lettuce, baby spinach leaves, very thinly sliced fennel, chicory, watercress or alfalfa sprouts.**

Per Serving:
Calories (kcal) 67.7
Protein (g) 4.1
Carbohydrates (g) 14.2
Total Sugars (g) 7.4
Dietary Fibre (g) 3.9
Fat (g) 0.4
Saturated Fat (g) 0.1

74% carbohydrate, GL: ●●●

warm hijiki salad with tofu

Serves 4 **Time taken:** 50 minutes

30g/1 oz Hijiki
250g/8^1/$_2$ oz Firm tofu, drained and cut into small squares (1 packet)
2 tsp Dark sesame oil
3 tbsp Tamari
1 tbsp Coconut oil
1 Garlic clove, finely chopped
2 Carrots, cut into julienne strips
4 sticks of Celery, cut into julienne strips
1 tbsp Rice vinegar or cider vinegar
1 tsp Brown rice syrup

1 Rinse the hijiki and soak in enough cold water to cover in a large bowl for 15-20 minutes. It will expand to 4-5 times its original volume. Drain, rinse and pat dry.

2 While the hijiki is soaking, marinate the tofu cubes in the sesame oil and one tablespoonful of the tamari.

3 Heat the coconut oil in a large non-stick frying pan or wok and stir fry the hijiki for 5 minutes. Add the garlic, carrot and celery and continue to stir fry for another couple of minutes. Add 200ml/7 fl oz water, the rest of the tamari, vinegar and brown rice syrup. Bring to the boil, then reduce the heat, cover and simmer for about 8 minutes, until the hijiki is tender but still has some bite. Drain well, reserving the cooking liquid, and keep warm.

4 Wipe out the pan and place over medium-high heat. Drain the tofu of its marinade and stir fry for a few minutes. Remove from the pan and keep warm.

5 Pour the cooking liquid from the hijiki back into the pan and reduce over a high heat until there is only a spoonful or two left. Spoon the hijiki salad on to 4 individual plates, pour over the reduced liquid and top with the tofu cubes. Serve the salad warm.

Note: Sea vegetables are such a nutritious food that we should try to include them frequently in our diet. They are full of minerals, especially calcium and iron. They are useful for people who are overweight as they add physical bulk to a meal yet are low in calories and fat. Their high fibre content makes them filling and therefore a useful part of a weight-loss diet. Because soybeans are very low GI, tofu is a good choice for diabetics, and an especially useful source of protein for vegetarians. 25g of the protein in soya, if eaten daily for 4 weeks, has been shown to decrease LDL (the 'bad' cholesterol) in people with raised blood cholesterol.

20% carbohydrate, GL: L ● ●

Hijiki is a Japanese seaweed that we can buy in this country dried in packets. Both Sanchi and Clearspring import it (see Useful Addresses). Hijiki looks like delicate black spaghetti, and makes a beautiful salad, the black contrasting with the orange carrot and pale green celery. You could easily double this recipe to have as a main course. It is a delicious introduction to tofu for those who have never tried it.

Per Serving:
Calories (kcal) 148.5
Protein (g) 9.6
Carbohydrates (g) 8.0
Total Sugars (g) 3.4
Dietary Fibre (g) 2.4
Fat (g) 9.6
Saturated Fat (g) 4.1

braised spring vegetables

This is a classic French dish. Since it's rarely possible to have these vegetables fresh all at the same time, it's perfectly acceptable to use frozen broad beans if necessary.

Serves 4 Time taken: 30 minutes

1 bunch **Radishes**
1 bunch **Spring onions**
20 **Baby carrots**
225g/8 oz (1/2 pound) **Courgettes**
6 **Asparagus spears**
1 **Little Gem lettuce**
200g/7 oz (1 cup) **Small fresh or frozen broad beans**
25g/1oz (2 tbsp) **Organic unsalted butter**
175ml/6 fl oz (3/4 cup) **Vegetable stock**
Sea salt and freshly ground black pepper
2 tbsp **Chopped fresh herbs, such as chives, parsley, tarragon and chervil**

1 Trim the radishes and spring onions. Scrape and trim the carrots: leave them whole if small enough, otherwise cut into batons. Cut the courgettes into batons, and the asparagus into lengths the same size as the carrots. Shred the lettuce finely.

2 Simmer the radishes in a small pan until tender, about 10 minutes, then drain and set aside. Simmer the broad beans in a separate pan – for 2 minutes if frozen, for about 5 minutes if fresh. Refresh in cold water. If they are small enough there is no need to skin them, which is a tiresome and time-consuming task. Set aside.

3 Put the carrots, butter and stock into a casserole. Bring to the boil, cover and simmer for 12 minutes. Add the courgettes and spring onions. Cover and cook for a further 3 minutes, then add the asparagus and cook for a further 3 minutes without the lid. Then add the broad beans, lettuce and radishes. Raise the heat enough to evaporate any remaining stock and lightly cook the lettuce, but don't let it change colour. Taste for seasoning, stir in the herbs and serve immediately.

Note: **All vegetables are good sources of potassium, the mineral we need to balance sodium in order to keep our blood pressure under control. This dish of braised vegetables supplies four times as much potassium as sodium (as long as you don't add any salt) and so it helps to redress the balance.**

Per Serving:
Calories (kcal) 131.6
Protein (g) 4.6
Carbohydrates (g) 16
Total Sugars (g) 5.1
Dietary Fibre (g) 4.9
Fat (g) 6.1
Saturated Fat (g) 3.7

47% carbohydrate, GL: L ● ●

kale with bagna cauda

Serves 4 **Time taken:** 10 minutes

500g/1lb Kale
1 tbsp Extra virgin olive oil
3 Garlic cloves, peeled and finely chopped
4 Anchovy fillets, finely chopped

1 Remove the hard stems from the kale and slice into 2.5cm/1" lengths. Slice the leaves into strips. Steam the stems and sliced leaves over hot water for 7-8 minutes or until just tender. Meanwhile, heat the oil in a small saucepan over low heat. Add the garlic and anchovy fillets and cook just until the garlic starts to change colour. Toss the steamed kale with the sauce and serve hot.

Note: Kale is a highly nutritious and rather neglected vegetable. It is the best source of magnesium and calcium in the vegetable world. It is also rich in potassium and folate, thiamine and vitamin B6. In addition, it is positively bristling with cancer-fighting phytochemicals and glucosinolates. Kale consumption has been linked with lower incidences of colon and bladder cancer.

I've taken some liberties with this recipe. Traditional Bagna Cauda is a Piedmontese hot sauce of butter, olive oil, garlic and anchovies into which you dip raw vegetables. I've taken out the butter and most of the oil, and used the sauce to jazz up plain steamed kale. Delicious and very more-ish, but note that this dish is quite high in sodium due to the anchovies.

Per Serving:
Calories (kcal) 87
Protein (g) 4.3
Carbohydrates (g) 9.7
Total Sugars (g) 1.8
Dietary Fibre (g) 4.2
Fat (g) 4.4
Saturated Fat (g) 0.7

40% carbohydrate, GL: Ⓛ ⚫ ⚫

gajar matar

This is a North Indian way with peas and carrots. It can be made with either fresh or frozen peas, so it's a useful winter staple vegetable dish that goes with Indian meals.

Serves 6 **Time taken:** 20 minutes

1 small Onion, peeled and roughly chopped
1 Garlic clove, peeled and roughly chopped
2.5cm/1" piece of Root ginger, peeled and chopped
60ml/2 fl oz (1/4 cup) Groundnut oil
1 tsp Cumin seeds
1 1/2 tsp Ground turmeric
340g/12 oz Carrots, diced
1 tsp Ground cumin
1 tsp Ground coriander
255g/9 oz (1 2/3 cups) Shelled fresh peas or frozen peas
1/4 tsp Chilli powder
4 tsp Pomegranate seeds (optional)
1/2 tsp Garam masala (see page 144)

1 Put the onion, garlic and ginger in the food processor and blend until finely chopped.

2 Heat the oil in a frying pan, then add the onion mixture and stir over medium heat until softened. Add the cumin seeds and turmeric. When the seeds are sizzling, add the carrots and stir fry for 2 minutes. Add the ground cumin and coriander and fry for a further 2 minutes. Stir in the peas and chilli powder. Add 4 tablespoons water (2 tablespoons if you are using frozen peas). Reduce the heat to low, add the pomegranate seeds, if using, and stir. Then cover the pan and simmer for 10 minutes, or until the vegetables are tender. Stir in the garam masala and serve hot.

Note: Fresh peas are a good source of vitamin C and they also supply iron, carotenes and the B vitamins. Few of these nutrients are reduced by freezing, so frozen peas are almost as nutritious as fresh. The pomegranate seeds boost the antioxidants in this dish, but they're not essential. They are credited with all sorts of health benefits, from reducing breast cancer risk to lowering the oxidation of LDL cholesterol.

Per Serving:
Calories (kcal) 226.4
Protein (g) 4.4
Carbohydrates (g) 21.0
Total Sugars (g) 8.8
Dietary Fibre (g) 6.7
Fat (g) 14.8
Saturated Fat (g) 2.3

36% carbohydrate, GL: ● Ⓜ ●

japanese stir-fry

Serves 4 **Time taken:** 15 minutes

1 tbsp **Sesame oil**
1 tbsp **Sake or dry sherry**
1 tbsp **Rice vinegar**
1 tsp **Concentrated apple juice**
1 tbsp **Water**
225g/8oz (1 cup) **Broccoli, cut into florets**
1 tbsp **Groundnut oil**
1cm/$^{1}/_{2}$" piece **Root ginger, peeled and grated**
225g/8 oz (2 cups) **Carrots, cut into 2.5cm/1" strips**
100g/3$^{1}/_{2}$ oz (1 cup) **Mushrooms, sliced**

1 For the sauce, mix together the sesame oil, sake or sherry, rice vinegar, apple juice and water.

2 Steam the broccoli for about 4 minutes, so that it is half cooked. Refresh in cold water to preserve the colour and then drain and set aside.

3 Heat the oil in a wok or large frying pan. Add the grated ginger and the carrots and stir fry for about 2-3 minutes. Add the mushrooms and stir fry for a further minute. Pour in the sauce mixture and bring to the boil, then reduce the heat. Cover and leave to simmer for about 3 minutes. Add the partially cooked broccoli and continue to cook for another 2-3 minutes until all the vegetables are cooked but still have some bite. Serve piping hot.

Note: Several of these mixed vegetable recipes contain broccoli. This is deliberate – not only is it easy and quick to prepare and cook, it's fast becoming the nation's favourite vegetable, and it is highly nutritious. The virtues of broccoli are too numerous to mention, but they include cancer-protective phytonutrients, vitamins C and E, calcium and iron. Purple sprouting broccoli is a special delicacy, at its best in the spring.

A very quick and easy stir-fry to serve with an oriental meal or with plainly cooked fish or meat. Feel free to vary the vegetables.

Per Serving:
Calories (kcal) 120.6
Protein (g) 2.4
Carbohydrates (g) 12.3
Total Sugars (g) 4.8
Dietary Fibre (g) 4.1
Fat (g) 7.5
Saturated Fat (g) 1.1

38% carbohydrate, GL: L ● ●

moghlai spinach

Serves 4 Time taken: 15 minutes

4 tbsp Extra virgin olive oil
3 medium Onions, peeled and finely sliced
2.5 cm/1" piece Fresh ginger root, peeled and grated
1 Fresh green chilli, deseeded and finely chopped
1.35 kg (3 lb) Spinach, washed and tough stalks removed
Sea salt and freshly ground black pepper
1/2 tsp Garam masala (see page 144)
4 tbsp Toasted cashew nuts, roughly chopped

1 Heat the olive oil in a large pan over medium heat. Sauté the onions, ginger and chilli, stirring constantly, until the onions are soft but not brown. Add the spinach, and season with salt and pepper. Stir once, then leave to cook for 3-4 minutes, until the spinach has cooked down. Before it loses its rich green colour, remove from the heat, stir once, add the garam masala and serve, garnished with the toasted chopped cashews.

Note: Spinach is an extremely rich source of magnesium, a key nutrient for people with diabetes, as it promotes healthy insulin production.

A quick way with spinach and good as part of an Indian meal. If I haven't got any garam masala to hand, I finish this with dukkah (see page 150) which gives the dish a nutty, spicy flavour.

Per Serving:
Calories (kcal) 272.5
Protein (g) 10.3
Carbohydrates (g) 21.2
Total Sugars (g) 5.3
Dietary Fibre (g) 7.8
Fat (g) 18.8
Saturated Fat (g) 2.9

29% carbohydrate, GL: L ● ●

spicy sweet potato purée

Serves 4 Time taken: 20 minutes

2 large Sweet potatoes (about 450g/1lb)
1 small Red chilli, seeded
Sea salt and freshly ground black pepper
Small bunch of fresh coriander, washed and roughly chopped
45g /1^{1}/$_{2}$ oz (3 tbsp) Organic unsalted butter
1 tbsp Extra virgin olive oil
2 tbsp Tamari

1 Peel the sweet potatoes and cut into large chunks. Put them in a saucepan with the chilli and enough cold water to cover, and season to taste. Bring to the boil over medium heat, then lower the heat and simmer for about 15 minutes until soft. Drain.

2 Tip the sweet potato and chilli into the blender. Add the coriander, butter, olive oil, and tamari and purée until smooth. Taste and adjust the seasoning, then reheat gently over low heat, stirring constantly. Serve as an accompaniment to meat or chicken dishes.

Note: Recent research studies on sweet potato have focused on two areas of health benefit. Firstly, some unique root storage proteins in sweet potatoes have been observed to have significant antioxidant capacities. Second is the recent classification of sweet potato as an 'antidiabetic' food because it has been shown to stabilise blood sugar levels and lower insulin resistance.

I've included this as a lower GI alternative to mashed potato. However, sweet potatoes have a GL of about 17, which is on the high side of medium, so they should only be eaten in moderate portions.

Per Serving:
Calories (kcal) 198.9
Protein (g) 3
Carbohydrates (g) 18.7
Total Sugars (g) 7.8
Dietary Fibre (g) 3
Fat (g) 12.6
Saturated Fat (g) 6.2

37% carbohydrate, GL: M

tempered cauliflower and chickpeas

This dish is Sri Lankan in origin, adapted to European tastes. You can replace the cauliflower with other vegetables such as broccoli, chard or spinach.

Serves 4-6 Time taken: 30 minutes

2 tsp Cumin seeds
1 tsp Coriander seeds
1/4 tsp Cardamom seeds
1 large Cauliflower, broken into small florets
2 tbsp Coconut oil
1 small Onion, peeled and finely chopped
2-3 Garlic cloves, peeled and crushed
1 Chilli, seeded and finely chopped
100ml/3 fl oz (1/3 cup) Coconut milk
400g can Chickpeas, drained and rinsed

1 First, grind the spices together in a pestle and mortar or electric grinder, and set aside. Steam the cauliflower florets over boiling water for about 5-6 minutes, so that they are still crunchy.

2 Heat the oil in a large frying pan or wok and fry the onion, garlic and chilli for a few minutes. Stir in the ground spices and cook for another five minutes over gentle heat, then stir in the steamed cauliflower. Stir fry for five minutes or so until the cauliflower is tender, then add the coconut milk and chickpeas. Mix thoroughly, cover and simmer for a few minutes. Serve as an accompaniment to meat or fish dishes.

Note: **Cauliflower, being a member of the Cruciferae family, has all the healing properties of cabbage or broccoli, but tends to be overlooked. It is a good source of folate. This is needed by the body to prevent levels of homocysteine from rising above normal. Raised levels of homocysteine are associated with heart disease.**

Per Serving:
Calories (kcal) 245.3
Protein (g) 9.2
Carbohydrates (g) 25.3
Total Sugars (g) 1.7
Dietary Fibre (g) 8.7
Fat (g) 13.8
Saturated Fat (g) 10.5

33% carbohydrate, GL: M

desserts and baking

The rosewater lends an exotic perfume to this fruit salad. If the fruits are all ripe, you will not notice the absence of sugar or other sweeteners.

scented tropical fruit salad

Serves 6 **Time taken:** 15 minutes plus chilling time

150ml/5 fl oz (2/3 cup) Apple juice
2 Limes
3 Cardamom pods
1 small bunch Fresh mint
3 tsp Rosewater
400g/14 oz Fresh pineapple (about half a pineapple)
1 Pink grapefruit
18 Lychees, fresh or canned
1 Papaya
1 Mango

1 Put the apple juice in a small pan. With a vegetable peeler, remove three broad strips of rind from the limes and add to the apple juice. Juice the limes and set aside. Bruise the cardamom pods with a rolling pin but don't pulverise them – you don't want to destroy the pods themselves. Put into the apple juice. Heat to boiling point and boil for two minutes only. Remove from the heat. Add the mint leaves, retaining a few for garnish. Cover and leave to cool.

2 When cool, remove the mint and add the lime juice and rosewater.

3 Peel the pineapple, discard the core and cut the flesh into small chunks. Peel and segment the grapefruit. Peel and stone the lychees, if fresh. Peel and slice the papaya and mango into bite-sized pieces.

4 Put the fruit into a large glass serving bowl or six individual serving bowls, and strain over the scented apple juice. Serve chilled, garnished with the reserved mint leaves.

Note: Fruit is almost all carbohydrate, so should be treated with caution and eaten in small portions. Some of these fruits are high GI, although grapefruit is very low. It would be sensible to eat this only after a high protein main course such as grilled fish, poultry or meat.

Per Serving:
Calories (kcal) 135.1
Protein (g) 1.8
Carbohydrates (g) 35.0
Total Sugars (g) 23.9
Dietary Fibre (g) 4.1
Fat (g) 0.5
Saturated Fat (g) 0.1

92% carbohydrate, GL: ● ● **H**

spice-roasted nectarines with cashew cream

Serves 4 **Time taken:** 15 minutes

4 large, Firm nectarines
45g/1¹/₂ oz (3 tbsp) Organic unsalted butter
10 Black peppercorns, cracked
¹/₂ tsp Szechuan peppercorns
¹/₂ tsp Ground star anise
30g/1 oz (2 tbsp) Organic brown sugar
2 tbsp Kirsch or other liqueur (optional)
To serve: 1 recipe Cashew cream (see page 152)

1 Preheat the oven to 230°C/450°F/gas 8.

2 Peel the nectarines: nick the skin at the stalk end, then plunge them into a bowl of boiling water for a minute or two - this makes the skins easy to remove. Cut the nectarines in half and remove the stones. Place the halves in an ovenproof baking dish.

3 Melt the butter in a non-stick frying pan, add the spices and cook for 1 minute. Add the sugar and 100ml/3 fl oz/¹/₃ cup of water. Bring to the boil and cook until the mixture is a light caramel colour; then add the kirsch if using. Pour the syrup over the nectarines and place in the oven to roast for 5-6 minutes.

4 To serve, pour a pool of cashew cream in the centre of each plate, add two nectarine halves and pour over the pan syrup.

Note: The GI of nectarines doesn't seem to have been tested, but since both peaches and plums are low GI, and a nectarine is a hybrid of both, it would follow that they are also low GI.

This recipe is a considerable adaptation of one by Paul Gayler, the executive chef of the Lanesborough Hotel in London, and an innovative creator of exquisite vegetarian recipes.

Per Serving:
Calories (kcal) 301.9
Protein (g) 4.9
Carbohydrates (g) 31.1
Total Sugars (g) 22.3
Dietary Fibre (g) 3.3
Fat (g) 17.7
Saturated Fat (g) 7.1

39% carbohydrate, GL: ● **M** ●

passion fruit pots de crème

This is unbelievably easy and really scrumptious with a tropical scent. Make sure you use really ripe passion fruit – their skins should be dry and wrinkled.

Serves 4 Time taken: 50 minutes

4 large Free-range eggs, beaten
3 tbsp Organic brown sugar
150ml/¹/₄ pint (²/₃ cup) Coconut milk
2 Passion fruit

1 Preheat the oven to 180°C/350°F/gas 4. Whisk together the eggs, sugar and coconut milk until smooth. Halve one passion fruit, scoop out the pulp and seeds and stir into the custard. Pour into 4 ramekins.

2 Put the ramekins in a roasting tin and pour boiling water into the tin to come three quarters of the way up the sides of the ramekins. Bake the custards for 40 minutes or until firm. Put the pulp and seeds from the second passion fruit on top and serve warm or cold.

Note: **Passion fruit have a low GI (30), are rich in vitamin C and a good source of vitamin A, iron and potassium.**

Per Serving:
Calories (kcal) 206.4
Protein (g) 7.2
Carbohydrates (g) 16.5
Total Sugars (g) 13
Dietary Fibre (g) 1.3
Fat (g) 12.8
Saturated Fat (g) 8.4

31% carbohydrate, GL: Ⓛ ⬤⬤

dried fruit pashka

Serves 4 Time taken: 15 minutes, plus overnight draining

340g/12 oz (1 1/2 cups) Cottage cheese
170g/6 oz (3/4 cup) Natural live yoghurt (see page 140)
2 tbsp Honey
1/2 tsp Pure vanilla extract
2 tbsp Candied peel, chopped
Grated rind of one orange
Grated rind of one lemon
2 tbsp Unblanched almonds, chopped
1 tbsp Raisins
1 Orange, for decoration

1 Drain any liquid from the cottage cheese. Place it in a sieve and, using a wooden spoon, rub it through the sieve into a bowl. Stir in the yoghurt, honey and vanilla extract. Then add the candied peel, the grated citrus rind, almonds and raisins, reserving a little of the citrus rind for decoration.

2 Line the flowerpot with the muslin, add the cheese mixture and press down firmly. Fold the muslin over the pudding and place a saucer with some weights on it on top. Put the pot on a saucer and refrigerate overnight. Any excess liquid will drip out at the hole in the bottom of the pot.

3 The next day, turn the pot upside down, turn out the pashka onto a serving plate and discard the muslin. Slice the whole orange and cut the slices in half. Surround the pashka with these and sprinkle it with the reserved grated orange and lemon peel.

Note: **This pudding has quite a lot of sugar – honey and raisins are both sources of simple sugars. This is to some extent balanced by the protein in the cottage cheese, but it still needs to be treated with care and eaten in small portions.**

Pashka is a traditional Russian dessert, usually made with double cream and raw egg whites and served at Easter. My version uses strained cottage cheese and yoghurt, thus cutting down on the saturated fat without sacrificing taste. You will need a clean clay flower pot and some clean muslin for this recipe.

Per Serving:
Calories (kcal) 190.8
Protein (g) 13.5
Carbohydrates (g) 22.0
Total Sugars (g) 16.2
Dietary Fibre (g) 1.6
Fat (g) 6.4
Saturated Fat (g) 2.9

44% carbohydrate, GL: **M**

Indian rice puddings are lighter than Western versions, but normally very sweet. In this recipe I've used brown basmati rice, cut down on the sugar and added some rosewater for an exotic touch. Sometimes saffron is added to kheer, which makes it a beautiful yellow colour. It's very rich, so you only need a small quantity.

Per Serving:
Calories (kcal) 178.9
Protein (g) 8.1
Carbohydrates (g) 24.2
Total Sugars (g) 12.1
Dietary Fibre (g) 1.5
Fat (g) 6
Saturated Fat (g) 2.7

kheer

Serves 4 **Time taken:** 15 minutes

60g/2 oz (1/4 cup) **Brown basmati rice**
450ml/16 fl oz (2 cups) **Water**
720ml/1 1/4 pints (3 1/4 cups) **Organic milk or dairy free alternative**
4 **Green cardamom pods**
1 **Cinnamon stick**
1 tbsp **Organic brown sugar (optional)**
2 tbsp **Flaked almonds**
1/4 tsp **Freshly grated nutmeg**
1 tbsp **Rosewater**
Freshly grated nutmeg for garnish

1 Rinse the rice thoroughly. Bring the water to a boil, throw in the rice and cook over medium heat for 10 minutes. Drain.

2 Bring the milk to a boil over medium heat together with two of the cardamom pods and the cinnamon stick. Add the rice, reduce the heat to low and cook for one hour, until the rice is soft and the milk is very thick. Stir occasionally at first and then constantly when the milk begins to thicken, during the last 10 minutes, to prevent the mixture from sticking to the bottom of the pan. Grind the seeds of the remaining two cardamom pods in a pestle and mortar and add to the rice, along with the sugar (if using), almonds and nutmeg. Cook for another 5 minutes, stirring constantly. Remove from the heat and discard the cinnamon stick and whole cardamom pods. Stir in the rosewater.

3 Serve warm or chilled in glass bowls with a little freshly grated nutmeg as garnish.

Note: If you are using rice milk or soya milk, which are usually sweetened with concentrated apple juice, you may find that you don't need any sugar at all.

53% carbohydrate, GL:

blueberry and tofu creams

Serves 4 Time taken: 10 minutes

250g/9 oz **Silken tofu**
60 ml /2 fl oz (1/4 cup) **Apple juice**
60ml /2 fl oz (1/4 cup) **Soya cream or coconut cream**
125g/41/2 oz (2/3 cup) **Blueberries**
To garnish: **Handful of blueberries**

1 Just put all the ingredients into the blender or food processor and blend until relatively smooth. A few bits of blueberry add a bit of texture so don't worry about those. Spoon into small bowls or dessert glasses and serve garnished with whole blueberries.

Note: **Using tofu like this is a great way to increase protein (and thus reduce the glycaemic load). Since it doesn't really taste of anything very much, it's a useful ingredient to add to any creamy blend. For example, you could sneak some into the tropical banana freeze on page 130 or the cashew cream on page 152.**

This is the easiest pudding ever, and it has a relatively good protein profile due to the presence of tofu.
As well as being a dessert, this is a lovely breakfast because it's so quick, tasty and nutritionally balanced.

Per Serving:
Calories (kcal) 74.1
Protein (g) 3.2
Carbohydrates (g) 9.2
Total Sugars (g) 5.7
Dietary Fibre (g) 0.8
Fat (g) 2.8
Saturated Fat (g) 0.2

49% carbohydrate, GL: L ● ●

tropical banana freeze

Serves 4 **Time taken:** 10 minutes plus 1 hour freezing

4 Bananas, peeled
1 tbsp Grated fresh, frozen or desiccated coconut
1 tbsp Sesame seeds
100ml/3 fl oz Coconut milk
1 tbsp Honey
1 Lime, juice only

1 Slice the bananas into 2.5cm/1" pieces, lay them on a baking tray and freeze until hard (at least one hour).

2 Dry fry the coconut and sesame seeds, stirring frequently, until browned.

3 Just before serving, take the bananas from the freezer and place in the blender with the coconut milk, honey and lime juice. Blend until smooth. Serve in small glass bowls, garnished with the toasted coconut and sesame seeds.

Note: The GL of a banana depends on the variety of banana, where it was grown, and most importantly, how ripe it is. Choose slightly underripe bananas and the GL can be as low as 11, and even the mean of 10 studies was only 12.

I've used honey in this and several of the other dessert recipes. It is a concentrated sugar, being composed of a combination of fructose and glucose, but it does contain some trace elements too, so I think it preferable to other 'natural' syrups on the market.

Per Serving:
Calories (kcal) 189.8
Protein (g) 2.3
Carbohydrates (g) 33.6
Total Sugars (g) 17.4
Dietary Fibre (g) 3.8
Fat (g) 7.2
Saturated Fat (g) 5.2

65% carbohydrate, GL: M

berry semifreddo

Serves 6 Time taken: 10 minutes plus freezing time

225g/8 oz (2 cups) Fresh blueberries
225g/8 oz (2 cups) Fresh raspberries
500g/1lb (2 cups) Fresh strawberries
175ml/6 fl oz (3/4 cup) Apple juice
450g/1lb (1 3/4 cups) Live natural yoghurt (see page 140)
Garnish: Mint leaves and whole berries

1 Prepare the berries: remove any stems, wash and rinse. Reserve a few berries for garnish. Place apple juice in a blender and add all the berries. Blend thoroughly, turn into a large mixing bowl and stir in the yoghurt.

2 Place in a shallow container and freeze for about one hour (or less if you were using frozen berries). Remove from the freezer and stir the mixture vigorously to break ice created over the top. The mixture should be served when it is partially frozen but still of a liquid consistency.

3 Ladle into bowls and garnish with mint leaves and the reserved whole berries.

Note: All berries are packed with nutrition, especially the darker coloured ones such as blueberries, which come top of the 'ORAC' scale. The ORAC rating of a food means its Oxygen Radical Absorbance Capacity - the ability to absorb the dangerous free radicals which are ultimately responsible for all cellular damage. Strawberries and raspberries are also in the top 10 foods on the ORAC scale.

'Semifreddo' is Italian for 'half cold'. This is a very simple mixture of berries and yoghurt which goes into the freezer for a short time so that it's about the same consistency as thick cream. Out of season, you could substitute unsweetened frozen fruits.

Per Serving:
Calories (kcal) 134.9
Protein (g) 5.6
Carbohydrates (g) 28.2
Total Sugars (g) 11.9
Dietary Fibre (g) 5.3
Fat (g) 1.7
Saturated Fat (g) 0.9

75% carbohydrate, GL: ● M ●

coconut and lime ice cream

I love cooking with coconut. This has a wonderfully tropical taste and reminds me of the Caribbean where
I cooked for some years. There is some honey in this ice cream, but its glycaemic effect should be moderated by the fat in the coconut and egg yolks.

Serves 6 **Time taken:** 15 minutes

4 Free-range egg yolks
1 heaped tsp Cornflour
2 tbsp Honey
400ml/14 fl oz (1 1/2 cups) Coconut milk
100ml/3 fl oz (1/3 cup) Coconut cream (or 2 x 50g sachets)
5 tbsp Desiccated coconut
2 Limes, grated zest and juice
To serve: Strips of toasted or dried coconut (optional)

1 Mix the egg yolks, cornflour and honey together in a bowl, then slowly add the coconut milk. Transfer to a saucepan, add the desiccated coconut and cook over a very low heat or in a double boiler, stirring constantly. The mixture must not be allowed to boil or the egg yolks will curdle. Cook until slightly thickened, then remove from the heat. Stir in the coconut cream, grated lime zest and lime juice. Taste to make sure the balance between coconut and lime is just right – you may not need all the lime juice. Cool to room temperature.

2 Churn the ice cream in an ice cream machine if you have one, following the manufacturer's instructions. Or you can freeze it in a shallow container, beating the mixture 3 or 4 times during the freezing process.

3 Take out of the freezer to soften before serving. Serve garnished with strips of toasted coconut if liked.

Note: Coconut, and particularly coconut oil, was implicated in raising cholesterol levels by some poorly conducted research in the 1950s, and it has taken a long time for it to shake off this bad reputation. In fact, 50% of the fatty acids it contains are in the form of a medium chain fatty acid called lauric acid. Lauric acid actually helps to regulate blood sugar. One of the contributing factors to the huge rise in diabetes in India is thought to be because people have abandoned coconut oil in favour of refined vegetable oils. So coconut, coconut cream and coconut oil are actually healthy foods for people with diabetes.

Per Serving:
Calories (kcal) 379
Protein (g) 5.3
Carbohydrates (g) 18.3
Total Sugars (g) 10.2
Dietary Fibre (g) 4.5
Fat (g) 34.2
Saturated Fat (g) 28.4

18% carbohydrate, GL: ●●●

muesli plum crumble

Serves 4 Time taken: 1 hour

450g/1lb Pumpkin seed and almond muesli (see page 29)
1 tsp Ground cinnamon
45g/1$^{1}/_{2}$ oz (3 tbsp) Organic unsalted butter
800g/1$^{3}/_{4}$ lbs Plums, halved and stoned
4-5 Star anise
1 tbsp Honey
4 tbsp Water
To serve: Natural yoghurt (see page 140) or cashew cream (see page 152)

1 Preheat the oven to 180°C/350°F/gas 4.

2 Mix together the muesli and cinnamon in a large bowl. Rub in the butter in small pieces.

3 Put the plums and star anise in a baking dish, and pour over the honey and water. Cover the plums with the crumble mixture, and press down so that there is no fruit showing through the crumble. Bake for 45 minutes or until the plums are tender. Serve hot with yoghurt or cashew cream.

Note: Try this crumble with other fruits, such as blackberry and apple, peaches or fresh apricots. I chose plums because they are low GI and often taste better cooked than raw.

If you are surprised to see a recipe for a traditional English pudding in a book for diabetics, think again. This recipe uses a low GI topping and contains plums, which are low GI, cinnamon, which is known to lower blood glucose, pumpkin seeds and walnuts.

Per Serving:
Calories (kcal) 339.8
Protein (g) 8.3
Carbohydrates (g) 43.2
Total Sugars (g) 23.7
Dietary Fibre (g) 7.1
Fat (g) 17.8
Saturated Fat (g) 6.6

47% carbohydrate, GL: ● **M** ●

baked apricot and blueberry squares

This is a typical American 'tray bake' but without the sugar. Instead, it relies for its sweetness on the fruit and the discreet addition of a banana.

Makes 24 squares **Time taken:** 1 hour 10 minutes

200g/7 oz **Unsulphured dried apricots, roughly chopped**
100ml/3 fl oz (1/3 cup) **Apple juice**
225g/8 oz (2 cups) **Ground almonds**
60g/2 oz (4 tbsp) **Flaked almonds**
45g/1 1/2 oz (3 tbsp) **Gluten-free flour**
2 tsp **Baking powder**
6 **Free-range eggs**
170g/6 oz (1 1/2 sticks) **Organic unsalted butter, softened**
1 **Banana, mashed**
1 **Lemon, juice and finely grated zest**
125g/4 1/2 oz (1 cup) **Fresh blueberries**

1 Put the apricots in a small pan with the apple juice. Bring to a gentle simmer and cook over low heat for a few minutes, then take off the heat and set aside.

2 Preheat the oven to 220°C/425°F/gas 7 and grease a deep sided 23 x 30cm/9" x 12" baking tin (I use a roasting tin for this).

3 Mix together the ground and flaked almonds, flour and baking powder in a large bowl. Beat together the eggs, butter, mashed banana, lemon zest and juice, and stir this mixture into the dry ingredients. Drain the apricots and stir into the mixture together with the blueberries, working quickly. Spoon the mixture into the prepared pan. Bake in the preheated oven for 25-30 minutes, or until a knife inserted into the middle of the cake comes out clean. If there is fruit on the top which looks as though it's burning, cover loosely with foil. Leave to cool in the tin, then cut into squares. Eat warm with cashew cream as a pudding, or serve at room temperature as a cake. This is best eaten the day it is made.

Note: I've chosen dried apricots and blueberries because they are both low GI, apricots are a very good source of potassium and blueberries are rich in antioxidants. But you could vary the recipe using other dried fruit such as chopped figs or dates, and substitute chopped eating apples, pears or raspberries.

Per Serving:
Calories (kcal) 178
Protein (g) 4.6
Carbohydrates (g) 11.7
Total Sugars (g) 2.3
Dietary Fibre (g) 2.3
Fat (g) 12.9
Saturated Fat (g) 4.4

26% carbohydrate, GL: M

orange and almond cake

Serves 8 Time taken: 3 hours 15 minutes

2 large Oranges
6 Free-range eggs
225g/8 oz (2 cups) Ground almonds
110g/4 oz (²/₃ cup) Organic brown sugar
1 tsp Baking powder

1 Wash and boil the whole, unpeeled oranges in a little water for 2 hours, or until very tender, topping up the water from time to time. This process can be carried out in a pressure cooker, in which case it will take 30 minutes. Drain and cool the oranges, remove the pips and reduce to a pulp in a food processor or by passing them through a sieve.

2 Preheat the oven to 200°C/400°F/gas 6. Grease and line an 20cm/8.5" springform cake tin.

3 Beat the eggs in a large bowl and fold in all the other ingredients, including the oranges. Turn into the prepared cake tin and bake for an hour. Test with a sharp knife or skewer – it will come out clean if the cake is done. If not, bake for a little longer. Cool and serve as a teatime cake, or as a dessert with yoghurt and soft fruit.

Note: **This cake has fantastic keeping qualities. Because of the high proportion of eggs and ground almonds, it doesn't seem to dry out. I keep it in the fridge and it seems to last for up to a week. If I'm serving it to non-diabetics, I add a thin glaze of icing made with icing sugar and fresh orange juice.**

This is a Sephardic Jewish cake from the Middle East, popularised by Claudia Roden. She tells us that cakes such as this, using almonds instead of flour, show Portuguese or Spanish influence due to the thousand years the Sephardic Jews spent in the Iberian peninsula. The lack of flour makes it ideal for the diabetic, but it does still contain sugar, so treat with caution.

Per Serving:
Calories (kcal) 293.4
Protein (g) 11.1
Carbohydrates (g) 25.5
Total Sugars (g) 19.4
Dietary Fibre (g) 4.4
Fat (g) 18.1
Saturated Fat (g) 2.3

33% carbohydrate, GL: ● M ●

turkish yoghurt and lemon cheesecake

Here I have adapted a classic Turkish cake, a cheesecake only in name as it does not contain any cheese. It does contain honey, and a little flour, but I've pared down the recipe so that it's a lot lower in carbohydrate than most cakes.

Serves 6 **Time taken:** 1hr 10 minutes

4 large Free-range eggs, separated
60g/2 oz (1/3 cup) Honey
3 heaped tbsp Plain or gluten-free flour
400g/14 oz (1 1/2 cups) Greek yoghurt
1 Unwaxed lemon, grated zest and juice

1 Preheat the oven to 180°C/350°F/gas 4. Grease a 23cm/9" round baking tin with butter.

2 Beat the egg yolks with the honey to a pale cream. Beat in the flour, then the yoghurt, lemon zest and juice.

3 Whisk the egg whites until stiff and then fold them into the yoghurt mixture using a metal spoon. Pour into the prepared baking tin and bake in the preheated oven for 50-60 minutes, until the top is brown. This cake will puff up like a soufflé for a short time, but will subside again. When it is cooked, turn it out onto a plate. The cake can be eaten warm or at room temperature, accompanied, if liked, with soft fruit.

Note: If your non-diabetic guests find the lemony taste a bit sharp, simply sift over some icing sugar to sweeten it for them. You can do this with any dessert which other people might find is not sweet enough.

Per Serving:
Calories (kcal) 138.8
Protein (g) 6.9
Carbohydrates (g) 15.1
Total Sugars (g) 10.9
Dietary Fibre (g) 0.3
Fat (g) 5.6
Saturated Fat (g) 2.5

44% carbohydrate, GL: ● Ⓜ ●

three minute spelt bread

Makes 1 loaf **Time taken:** 1 hour 15 minutes

500g/1lb 2 oz (3^1/$_2$ cups) Spelt flour
10g/3^1/$_2$ tsp Fast acting dried yeast (1^1/$_2$ sachets)
^{1}/$_2$ tsp Sea salt
50g/2 oz (^{1}/$_2$ cup) Sunflower seeds
50g/2 oz (^{1}/$_2$ cup) Linseeds
500ml/18 fl oz (2^1/$_4$ cups) Warm water

1 Preheat the oven to 200°C/400°F/gas 6.

2 Combine all the ingredients, adding the water last. Mix well and turn the dough into a greased 2lb loaf tin. Put straight into the preheated oven and bake for 50-60 minutes, or until nicely browned. Remove the loaf, turn it out of the tin and then return it to the oven without the tin for a further 5-10 minutes.

Note: Spelt bread has a medium GL of between 12 and 17 per serving. This loaf can be made successfully in a breadmaker, using 400ml water instead of 500ml.

This is a remarkably simple loaf that rivals the breadmaking machine for ease and speed, but don't expect it to rise as much as a kneaded loaf would. The recipe was developed by Sybille Wilkinson of Gilchesters Organic Farm in Northumberland (see Useful Addresses) using their own organic spelt. Many people who are intolerant of wheat find that they can tolerate spelt, which is an ancient form of wheat. True celiacs would have to avoid it, however.

Per Serving:
Calories (kcal) 136.8
Protein (g) 4.6
Carbohydrates (g) 21.7
Total Sugars (g) 0.1
Dietary Fibre (g) 4.1
Fat (g) 3.3
Saturated Fat (g) 0.3

64% carbohydrate, GL: (M)

These rolls, from Dan Lepard, the brilliant Australian baker, are made with cooked lentils which gives them an interesting taste and moist texture. The original recipe was rather complicated, so I've simplified it by using fast-acting yeast, which cuts down on the proving time.

Per Serving:
Calories (kcal) 104.7
Protein (g) 5.8
Carbohydrates (g) 21.0
Total Sugars (g) 0.6
Dietary Fibre (g) 3.2
Fat (g) 0.3
Saturated Fat (g) 0

lentil rolls

Makes 16 rolls **Time taken:** 2$^1/_2$ hours

200g/7 oz (1 cup) Puy lentils
2$^1/_2$ tsp Fast acting dried yeast (1 sachet)
100ml/3$^1/_2$ fl oz (scant $^1/_2$ cup) Water at 20°C
225g/8 oz (1$^1/_2$ cups) Strong white flour
60g/2 oz ($^1/_3$ cup) Rye flour
1 tsp Sea salt

1 First, cook the lentils in water to cover for about 30 minutes, until soft. Drain and allow to cool. You should now have about 450g/1lb/3 cups of cooked lentils.

2 In a large bowl combine the cooked lentils with all the other ingredients. Mix everything together until you have a sticky dough, then turn out the dough onto a lightly floured work surface and knead for about 10 minutes, until the dough feels smooth and silky.

3 Roll the dough into a sheet measuring 25 x 20cm/10" x 8". Lay the dough on a tray lined with a cloth dusted with flour, cover with another cloth and leave in a warm place for an hour, until the dough has almost doubled in thickness.

4 Preheat the oven to 200°C/400°F/gas 6. Uncover the dough and cut into 16 squares. Carefully lift the squares up and place them on a baking tray dusted with flour. Bake in the preheated oven for 25 minutes, or until the rolls are pale brown and feel light.

Note: For the diabetic, the inclusion of a high protein and low GI ingredient like lentils means that the overall effect on blood sugar of these rolls is less dramatic than that of other breads. They also seem to keep very well, as the addition of lentils keep the rolls moist without any added fat.

76% carbohydrate, GL: ● M ●

miscellaneous

yoghurt

It's easy and satisfying to make your own yoghurt, and the result is less acidic than commercial yoghurts. Yoghurt, which is much easier to digest than milk or cream, is a staple food of many cuisines, particularly in the Middle East and the Indian subcontinent, and I have used it in many recipes in this book. It is important that the first batch is made with live yoghurt, as it contains the lactobacilli essential for fermenting the milk. Thereafter you can use your own yoghurt as a starter.

Makes 600ml/1 pint/2¹/₂ cups **Time taken:** 15 minutes plus 12 hours fermenting

600ml/1 pt (2¹/₂ cups) Organic whole milk
1 tbsp Natural live yoghurt

1 Bring the milk to the boil in a scrupulously clean saucepan. Cool to blood heat (37°C/98.6°F). Add the yoghurt to the milk and mix thoroughly. Pour the mixture into a clean vacuum flask and screw the top down securely. Leave the flask to stand for at least 12 hours.

2 Alternatively, pour the mixture into a clean shallow dish, cover it with a warmed plate and wrap in a towel. Leave in a warm place, such as an airing cupboard, for at least 12 hours.

Note: Because invading bacteria and variations in temperature can change the character of your yoghurt, you may prefer to invest in a yoghurt maker which does the job for you. Lakeland (see Useful Addresses) stocks two – one that relies on electricity and one that does not.

Per Serving:
Calories (kcal) 61.6
Protein (g) 3.5
Carbohydrates (g) 4.7
Total Sugars (g) 4.7
Dietary Fibre (g) 0
Fat (g) 3.3
Saturated Fat (g) 2.1

30% carbohydrate, GL: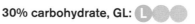

labneh

Makes approx 8 balls **Time taken:** 5 minutes plus 12 hours draining

600ml/1 pt (2$^{1}/_{2}$ cups) **Natural live yoghurt (see previous page)**
$^{1}/_{2}$ tsp **Sea salt**
1 tbsp **Extra virgin olive oil**
1 tbsp **Paprika**

1 Spoon the yoghurt into a sieve or colander lined with a piece of muslin that has been wrung out in water. Allow it to drain overnight in the fridge. The next day, discard the whey. The solid curds can be used without further preparation in recipes. Traditionally, it is rolled into small balls, and sprinkled with olive oil and paprika.

Note: The labneh balls can be preserved in olive oil. Fill a preserving jar with olive oil up to one third, then fill it up with labneh balls. Add oil as you go. When the jar is full, the balls should be covered with about 1cm/$^{1}/_{2}$" of oil. As long as they are always submerged in oil, the labneh balls will keep several months in this way, though they taste more and more sour as time goes on.

Labneh is a kind of yoghurt cheese eaten throughout the Middle East.

Per Serving:
Calories (kcal) 122.4
Protein (g) 7.5
Carbohydrates (g) 10.8
Total Sugars (g) 0.2
Dietary Fibre (g) 0.9
Fat (g) 5.6
Saturated Fat (g) 0.9

35% carbohydrate, GL: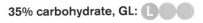

paneer

Paneer, the Indian 'cottage cheese', is made by coagulating milk with lemon juice. It is not worth making a small quantity: although this recipe starts off with a large quantity of milk, it only makes about 500g/1lb of paneer.
But it's much nicer than the commercial paneer you can buy, being softer and less rubbery.

Makes 500g/1lb **Time taken:** 15 minutes plus 12 hours draining

3 litres/5^1/$_4$ pts (13 cups) Organic whole milk
6 tbsp (7 tbsp) Strained lemon juice

1 Bring the milk to the boil in a large heavy-based saucepan, stirring. Reduce the heat and stir in the lemon juice, and cook for a few seconds until large curds start to form. Take off the heat and shake the pan to encourage curd formation. You may need to put it back on the heat for a minute or two to achieve this.

2 Line a colander with muslin. Carefully pour off the liquid whey and collect the curds in the muslin-lined colander. Twist the corners of the muslin together to form a bag, forcing the whey out. Then hold the bag under running water to wash any remaining whey off the outside of the bag, twisting it as you do so. Now suspend the bag over a bowl overnight in the fridge so that the weight of the curds forces out more liquid. Next day, put the bag on a plate and press it with a heavy weight to form a firm block. The paneer is now ready to use.

Per Serving:
Calories (kcal) 250.4
Protein (g) 12.7
Carbohydrates (g) 19
Total Sugars (g) 18.3
Dietary Fibre (g) 0
Fat (g) 14.2
Saturated Fat (g) 8.8

27% carbohydrate, GL: L ● ●

cucumber and mint raita

Serves 4 Time taken: 5 minutes

425ml/³/₄ pt (scant 2 cups) Natural live yoghurt (see page 140)
15cm/6" piece Cucumber, peeled and cut into 2cm/³/₄ inch cubes
2 tbsp (4 tbsp) Fresh mint leaves, finely chopped
³/₄ tsp Ground cumin seeds, roasted or dry fried
¹/₄ tsp Cayenne pepper
Sea salt and freshly ground black pepper to taste
Fresh mint leaves, for garnish

1 Put the yoghurt in a large bowl and stir. Add the cucumber, chopped mint, cumin seeds, cayenne pepper (if liked) and season to taste. Garnish with fresh mint leaves.

Note: Mint was deemed 'profitable to the stomach' by seventeenth century herbalist Nicholas Culpeper, and yoghurt has long been credited with improving gastro-intestinal health because of the beneficial bacteria it contains, so this combination is undoubtedly good for the digestion. Cucumbers are composed mainly of water, but are also credited with diuretic properties.

This is a classic Indian side dish. A yoghurt dish is served with almost every Indian meal as a contrast to hot and spicy dishes. You can vary the vegetables, using tomatoes, onions, grated carrots or even beetroot.

Per Serving:
Calories (kcal) 10.3
Protein (g) 0.7
Carbohydrates (g) 2
Total Sugars (g) 0.4
Dietary Fibre (g) 1
Fat (g) 0.2
Saturated Fat (g) 0

65% carbohydrate, GL: L

garam masala

Makes 3 tablespoons **Time taken:** 5 minutes

8 Cardamom pods
2 Cassia leaves or bay leaves
1 tsp Black peppercorns
2 tsp Cumin seeds
2 tsp Coriander seeds
5cm/2" piece of Cinnamon stick
1 tsp Whole cloves

1 Remove the seeds from the cardamom pods. Break the bay leaves into small pieces. Put them in a spice grinder or pestle and mortar with the remaining spices and grind to a fine powder. Store in a small airtight container.

Garam Masala means 'warming spice mix' and is designed to add flavour, rather than heat, at the end of the cooking process. It is often used to finish a dish.

Per Serving:
Calories (kcal) 27.9
Protein (g) 0.9
Carbohydrates (g) 5.6
Total Sugars (g) 0.1
Dietary Fibre (g) 2.9
Fat (g) 0.8
Saturated Fat (g) 0.1

67% carbohydrate, GL: L ● ●

mexican salsa picante

Serves 6 **Time taken:** 20 minutes

450g/1 lb Tomatoes, peeled and seeded
1 Onion, peeled and chopped
1 Clove garlic, peeled and chopped
1-2 Jalapeno or other hot chillies, peeled and seeded and roughly chopped
1 tbsp Extra virgin olive oil
$1/2$ tsp Sea salt

1 Put the tomatoes, onion, garlic and chillies in the blender or food processor. Blend just until the tomatoes are chopped small, but not puréed. Heat the oil in a medium saucepan and add the tomato mixture and salt. Bring to the boil, reduce the heat and simmer uncovered for about 10 minutes, until the sauce is a little reduced.

A classic spicy tomato sauce that can be used as an accompaniment to Mexican dishes, or to liven up beans, grains and plain steamed vegetables.

Per Serving:
Calories (kcal) 42.95
Protein (g) 0.99
Carbohydrates (g) 4.92
Dietary Fibre (g) 0.82
Fat (g) 2.46
Saturated Fat (g) 0.34

43% carbohydrate, GL: 🅛⬤⬤

This is a relatively mild fresh chutney that can be used to accompany any Indian dishes.

coconut chutney

Serves 4 Time taken: 25 minutes

90g/3 oz (1 cup) Grated fresh coconut
1 small Green chilli, chopped
1 tsp Grated fresh ginger root
1 tbsp Roasted chana dahl, optional
Sea salt to taste
For the tempering: **1 tsp Groundnut oil**
1/2 tsp Mustard seeds
1 Red chilli, broken into pieces
2-3 Curry leaves

1 Put the coconut, green chilli, ginger, roasted chana dahl and salt in a blender with a little water and grind to make a fine paste. Keep aside.

2 Prepare the tempering by heating the oil and adding the mustard seeds, red chilli and curry leaves and stirring till the mustard seeds crackle. Pour this tempering over the chutney and mix well.

3 Refrigerate and use as required.

Per Serving:
Calories (kcal) 114.4
Protein (g) 2.2
Carbohydrates (g) 7.8
Total Sugars (g) 2.6
Dietary Fibre (g) 2.4
Fat (g) 9
Saturated Fat (g) 6.9

26% carbohydrate, GL: L ● ●

harissa

Makes approx 450g/1lb, serves 12 **Time taken:** 15 minutes

3 Red peppers
1 tbsp Tomato purée
1 tbsp Ground coriander
1 tsp Saffron threads
10 small Green chillies, stalks removed and deseeded
1 tsp Sea salt
1 tsp Cayenne pepper

1 Roast or grill the peppers until their skins are charred. Leave to cool, then skin, deseed and chop roughly. Put into the blender with all the other ingredients and blend until relatively smooth. This is also good mixed with mayonnaise to make rouille, the fiery accompaniment to French fish soup and bouillabaisse.

This sauce comes from North Africa and is available in small tins from shops and supermarkets. This is my version which is a bit more aromatic than the bought versions, but equally fierce.
The heat of your chillies will determine the heat of the finished sauce.
Use fewer chillies if yours are very hot. This makes quite a large amount, but it keeps well in the fridge, covered with a layer of olive oil.

Per Serving:
Calories (kcal) 13.8
Protein (g) 0.6
Carbohydrates (g) 3.2
Total Sugars (g) 1
Dietary Fibre (g) 0.6
Fat (g) 0.1
Saturated Fat (g) 0

80% carbohydrate, GL: L ● ●

red pepper chutney

Serves 4 **Time taken:** 5 minutes

2 Red peppers, deseeded and roughly chopped
6 Dried red chillies
2 tbsp Cumin seeds
1 Lemon, juice only
Sea salt to taste

1 Whizz all the ingredients in the blender until smooth. Allow 30 minutes before serving to allow the flavours to blend together.

This chutney, with its wonderful bright red colour only keeps for a couple of days in the fridge, but it is so quick to make you can just whizz it up when you need it.

Per Serving:
Calories (kcal) 42.1
Protein (g) 1.6
Carbohydrates (g) 7.9
Total Sugars (g) 0.9
Dietary Fibre (g) 2.3
Fat (g) 1.7
Saturated Fat (g) 0.2

59% carbohydrate, GL: ●●●

kisir

Serves 10 **Time taken:** 25 minutes

110g/4 oz (1 cup) Shelled walnuts
6 Spring onions
4 Pickled Turkish chillies, or Spanish piquillo peppers
Small bunch of mint
Small bunch of dill
Small bunch of flat leaf parsley
1/2 Lemon, juice only
1 tbsp Tomato purée
2 tbsp Extra virgin olive oil
Sea salt and freshly ground black pepper

1 Preheat the oven to 180°C/350°F/gas 4.

2 Place the walnuts on a baking tray and roast for 15 minutes, stirring from time to time. While still hot, tip the nuts into a sieve or colander and shake out as much of the skins as possible. Cool, then chop roughly. Set the chopped nuts aside.

3 Trim and slice the spring onions finely. Chop the chillies or peppers and mix them and the onions into the chopped walnuts. Chop the herbs and add to the mixture. Mix together the lemon juice, tomato purée and olive oil and stir into the mixture. Season to taste and serve as a condiment or over lettuce.

This is a cracked wheat salad from Turkey, without the wheat. You can sprinkle it on anything. It is sometimes served on a plain lettuce salad. If you can't find pickled chillies or piquillo peppers, two roasted red peppers would make a good substitute.

Per Serving:
Calories (kcal) 117.2
Protein (g) 2.8
Carbohydrates (g) 5.7
Total Sugars (g) 1.2
Dietary Fibre (g) 2.3
Fat (g) 10.2
Saturated Fat (g) 1.1

18% carbohydrate, GL: L ● ●

This is an Egyptian seasoning mix. It should be crushed rather than ground into a powder and is normally eaten sprinkled on bread which has been dipped in olive oil. I find it quite addictive, and use it as a condiment on practically everything – tossed into brown rice, sprinkled on steamed vegetables or salad, or used as a coating on grilled chicken or fish. I have tried making dukkah with several different nuts, but this is my current favourite.

Per Serving:
Calories (kcal) 87.8
Protein (g) 2.7
Carbohydrates (g) 5.1
Total Sugars (g) 0.4
Dietary Fibre (g) 3.1
Fat (g) 7.9
Saturated Fat (g) 0.7

dukkah

Makes approx. 16 servings **Time taken:** 20 minutes

110g/4 oz (²/₃ cup) **Blanched almonds**
75g/2¹/₂ oz (¹/₂ cup) **Unhulled sesame seeds**
60g/2 oz (4 tbsp) **Coriander seeds**
30g/1 oz (2 tbsp) **Cumin**
1¹/₂ tsp **Sea salt**
¹/₂ tsp **Freshly ground black pepper**

1 Preheat the oven to 200°C/400°F/gas 6.

2 Spread the nuts out on a baking tray and roast until starting to brown (5-10 minutes), stirring from time to time. Leave to cool in a large bowl. Meanwhile, dry fry the sesame seeds in a cast-iron pan over medium heat until they pop (have a lid handy in case they threaten to jump out of the pan). Tip into the bowl of almonds and repeat with the coriander seeds, then the cumin seeds, toasting them until they release their fragrance. Add salt and pepper. Leave to cool, then crush in a pestle and mortar or in an electric nut grinder, in batches. Do this very briefly as you do not want the oils from the nuts and seeds to turn the whole thing into a paste. Stored in screw top jars this will keep for a long time.

Note: If you don't feel like making your own dukkah, Seasoned Pioneers do a very good ready-made mix. See Useful Addresses for details.

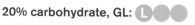

20% carbohydrate, GL:

preserved lemons

Makes 20 **Time taken:** 10 minutes plus 5 weeks standing time

20-24 Small thin-skinned lemons
30g/1 oz (1/4 cup) Coarse sea salt

These are an integral part of North African cooking.

1 Quarter 20 of the lemons, but don't cut all the way through – leave the slices attached at one end. Sprinkle a pinch of salt in the bottom of a large, earthenware or glass container (a large Kilner jar would be ideal for this) and another few pinches on each of the lemons. Pack the lemons into the container until they are crushed sufficiently to be submerged in their own juice. If they don't produce enough juice themselves, you may need to squeeze 2-4 more lemons to obtain sufficient juice. Cover with a lid or plate and leave in a cool place for 4 days.

2 On the fifth day, stir the lemons, and cover tightly with two or three layers of clingfilm, fastening with a rubber band. If you are using a Kilner jar, this is the time to seal it with the rubber gasket in place.

3 Leave the lemons undisturbed for at least a month. To use, rinse in cold water before adding to a recipe.

Per Serving:
Calories (kcal) 15
Protein (g) 0
Carbohydrates (g) 5
Total Sugars (g) 1
Dietary Fibre (g) 1
Fat (g) 0
Saturated Fat (g) 0

100% carbohydrate, GL: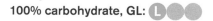

151

This is a useful sweet sauce to serve with desserts. Cashews work better than other nuts because of their relatively high carbohydrate content, and that makes the resulting cream sweeter and smoother than that made with other nuts such as almonds or walnuts. However, there's not enough carbohydrate in cashews to make you avoid them.

cashew cream

Serves 4 Time taken: 10 minutes

110g/4 oz ($^2/_3$ cup) Raw cashew nuts
120ml/4 fl oz ($^1/_2$ cup) Water
A few drops vanilla extract

1 Put the cashew nuts in the blender. Blend until pulverised, then pour in the water slowly with the machine running, until the mixture forms a thick cream. Finally, stir in the vanilla. The mixture will thicken on standing.

Per Serving:
Calories (kcal) 157.2
Protein (g) 5
Carbohydrates (g) 7.5
Total Sugars (g) 1.7
Dietary Fibre (g) 0.9
Fat (g) 12.9
Saturated Fat (g) 2.3

18% carbohydrate, GL: L ● ●

spicy masala chai

Serves 4 Time taken: 20 minutes

1 cm/¹/₂" piece Fresh ginger root, peeled and finely sliced
6 Cardamom pods, bruised with the back of a knife
1 Cinnamon stick
5 Whole cloves
600ml/1 pint (2¹/₂ cups) Water

1 Put all the ingredients in a large saucepan and bring to the boil. Lower the heat and simmer for 10-15 minutes. Strain and serve. This can be left to cool and reheated later, when the flavour is even more pronounced.

2 Another way to make this is to grind the cardamom seeds, cinnamon and cloves together first, before adding to the water with the ginger.

Chai means tea in many Asian languages. The word comes from cha, the Chinese word for tea. Masala is an Indian word meaning any spice blend. Masala chai is usually a brew of black tea with spices, sugar and milk, but this is a version without the tea. It's very warming on a cold night, or if you have a cold coming on.

Per Serving:
Calories (kcal) 10.2
Protein (g) 0.2
Carbohydrates (g) 2.2
Total Sugars (g) 0
Dietary Fibre (g) 1.1
Fat (g) 0.1
Saturated Fat (g) 0

83% carbohydrate, GL: L●●

153

salt lassi

This Indian yoghurt drink can be served alongside Indian dishes. Its protein content will help to balance the carbohydrate in rice and other grains.

Serves 4 Time taken: 10 minutes

1 tsp Cumin seeds
625ml/22 fl oz (2³/4 cups) Thick natural yoghurt
¹/2 tsp Sea salt

1 Dry roast the cumin seeds in a small pan over low heat until aromatic.

2 Reserve a few seeds for garnish, and put the rest into the blender with the yoghurt, salt and 300ml/¹/2 pint/1¹/4 cups water. Garnish with the reserved cumin seeds and serve at once.

Note: If you would like the lassi to be really ice-cold, replace a little of the water with ice cubes.

Per Serving:
Calories (kcal) 100.7
Protein (g) 5.7
Carbohydrates (g) 7.8
Total Sugars (g) 7.6
Dietary Fibre (g) 0.1
Fat (g) 5.4
Saturated Fat (g) 3.4

30% carbohydrate, GL: L ● ●

nut milk

Makes approx 400ml/12 fl oz/1³/₄ cups **Time taken:** 15 minutes

70g/2¹/₂ oz (¹/₂ cup) Nuts, such as almonds, Brazil nuts, walnuts, cashews or pecans
450ml/16 fl oz (2 cups) water
¹/₂ Banana (optional)

1 Put the nuts into a blender or food processor and process until ground. Add 120ml/
4 fl oz/¹/₂ cup of water and process at low speed for a few seconds, then increase the
speed. Blend for 2 minutes, then add the rest of the water, and the banana if using,
and blend again. Strain through a sieve, discarding the nut meal. The resulting milk is
quite grainy, so you may opt to strain it through muslin for a finer milk.

Milk can be made from almost any nuts, and makes a very nutritious and digestible alternative to dairy milk. I usually use blanched almonds, which I think make the best tasting milk, and I don't normally add any banana, but have done so here to appease those who prefer a sweeter milk.

Per Serving:
Calories (kcal) 79.3
Protein (g) 2.8
Carbohydrates (g) 4.7
Total Sugars (g) 1.8
Dietary Fibre (g) 1.5
Fat (g) 6.2
Saturated Fat (g) 0.5

22% carbohydrate, GL: L ● ●

diabetic menus from around the world

Use these menus to take a tour round the world, spending a day in each country eating diabetic-friendly dishes.

Country	Breakfast	Light Meal	Snack	Main meal	Carbohydrate & Glycaemic Load
Britain	Fresh raspberry porridge Nut milk	Beetroot and red cabbage soup with lentil rolls	Baked apricot and blueberry squares	Herring with mustard sauce Braised spring vegetables Fresh fruit	128g carbs Medium GL
France	Pipérade Fresh berries	Provençal tomato soup with basil and goat's cheese dumplings, lentil rolls	Chocolate petits fours	Navarin of lamb Steamed vegetables Passion fruit pots de crème	103g carbs Medium GL
Spain and the Mediterranean	Tortilla paisana Fresh fruit	Mediterranean roasted vegetables with beans	Toasted almonds	Roast sea bream with romesco sauce, steamed vegetables Spanish fig roll	110g carbs Medium GL
Turkey and Greece	Cornmeal Turkish-style	Greek courgette cakes with salad	Htipiti with raw vegetables	Fassolada Turkish yoghurt and lemon cheesecake	124g carbs Medium GL
Middle East	Iranian herb kuku	Barley and saffron soup	Aubergine dip, oat cakes	Tagine of lamb with apricots and preserved lemons Orange and almond cake	99g carbs Low/medium GL
India	Mango lassi Plain omelette	Indian stir-fry salad	Quick soya dhosas	Chana dahl with coconut and whole spices Cinnamon rice	162 g carbs Medium/high GL

Country	Breakfast	Light Meal	Snack	Main meal	Carbohydrate & Glycaemic Load
Thailand and Vietnam	Kao tom	Thai salad of prawns and grapefruit	Thai fish cakes with sweet and sour cucumber sauce	Chiang mai chicken curry, Vietnamese table salad Coconut and lime ice cream	109g carbs Low GL
Far East	Korean mung bean pancakes	Fragrant and hot prawns with green tea Brown rice	Tofu and coriander cakes	Aromatic five spice trout Japanese stir-fried vegetables Tropical banana freeze	132g carbs Medium GL
Mexico and Peru	Huevos rancheros with corn tortillas	Peruvian quinoa soup	Guacamole with raw vegetables	Pollo almendrado verde, brown rice, salad Scented tropical fruit salad	133g carbs Medium GL

shopping list

Vegetables – all vegetables, but cooked root vegetables in moderation only. Emphasise:

Beansprouts
Beetroot and beetroot greens (raw)
Broccoli
Cabbage
Celery
Chicory
Chinese cabbage
Courgettes
Garlic
Green beans
Jerusalem artichokes
Kale
Mushrooms
Olives
Onions
Peas, fresh or frozen
Peppers
Radishes
Sea vegetables
Spinach
Sweet potatoes
Sweetcorn
Tomatoes

Frozen vegetables are sometimes a better choice than 'fresh'

Whole Grains

Amaranth
Brown rice
Buckwheat
Buckwheat pasta (soba)
Nature's Path cereals such as Mesa Sunrise,
    Millet Flakes etc
Organic oat flakes, oat groats and oat bran
Pearl barley, pot barley
Polenta
Quinoa
Wholemeal pastas (any kind)

Fruits, emphasise:

Apples
Apricots
Avocados
Berries, eg blueberries, raspberries and strawberries
Cherries
Grapefruit
Grapes
Nectarines
Peaches
Pears
Plums

Dried fruit in moderation, such as:

Unsulphured apricots
Dried figs
Prunes

Protein Foods

Oily fish such as wild or organic salmon, mackerel,
  sea bass, herrings, trout, anchovies
White fish such as cod, haddock, plaice etc
Chicken, duck and guinea fowl (without skin)
Rabbit
Eggs, free-range and organic
Lean meat, all visible fat removed
Some cheeses, especially sheep's and goat's milk
  cheeses

Flour

Barley flour
Brown rice flour
Buckwheat flour
Chick pea flour
Gluten-free flour such as Dove's Farm
Stone-ground organic wholemeal, rye and spelt flour

Pulses, any kind such as

Black beans
Butterbeans
Chana dal
Chickpeas
Haricot beans
Kidney beans
Lentils, red, green and Puy
Soya beans and soya products such as tofu

Fats and Oils

Cold pressed extra virgin olive oil
Organic coconut oil
Groundnut oil for high temperature stir-frying
Butter in moderation
Flaxseed oil, walnut oil, avocado oil, pumpkin seed oil
  for salads

Spices - include

Cinnamon
Fenugreek seed
Ginger
Juniper berries

Beverages

Water
Vegetable juices
Fruit juices only if diluted (apple juice is best)
Red wine in moderation with food
Herbal teas, Green tea, black tea
Coffee, dandelion coffee

Sweeteners – minimal use only

Apple juice
Concentrated apple juice (Meridian)
Honey

Nuts and seeds, raw

Flaxseed (linseed)
Pumpkin seed
Sesame seeds
Sunflower seeds
Almonds
Brazil nuts
Walnuts
Nut and seed butters eg almond, hazelnut, tahini

shopping list

Dairy products (if using)

Organic natural live yoghurt
Cottage cheese
Occasional use of Parmesan and goat's/sheep's cheese

Optional milk alternatives

Soya milk
Rice Dream
Oat milk
Coconut milk

Bread alternatives

Rye bread (100% is best)
Rye crackers
Barley bread
Burgen Soya and Linseed bread (low GI)
Oatcakes
Doves Farm gluten-free savoury biscuits

Seasonings

Miso, both brown and white
Tamari/Shoyu (naturally brewed soy sauce)
Sea salt or low sodium salt
Fresh herbs of all kinds

Convenience Foods

Tinned beans – any kind
Sardines or pilchards in olive oil
Tomatoes – tinned/paste/dried/salsa
Hummus
Marinated tofu etc
Sugar free jams – Whole Earth

Food Equipment

Grinder – for nuts and seeds
Food processor
Food juicer for vegetable juices

the glycaemic index and glycaemic load

This is an extract of the latest tables available, which were published in 2002. Not all foods have been tested, and for reasons of space I have limited the extract here to more commonly used foods. The GI in these tables is based on an assumption that pure glucose has a GI of 100. Please note the following:

- Low GI is below 35 (NOT, as some authorities state, below 55)
- Medium GI is between 35 and 50
- High GI is above 50
- Low GL is below 10, medium GL is between 11 and 19, and high GL is 20 and above.
- Look for carbohydrate foods that are both low GI and low GL.

Food	GI Glucose	GL
BAKERY PRODUCTS		
Sponge cake, plain	46	16.6
Croissant	67	17.5
Crumpet	69	13.1
Doughnut	76	17.4
Pastry	59	15.4
BEVERAGES		
Cola soft drink	53	13.9
Orange soft drink	68	22.8
Sparkling glucose drink	95	39.7
Lemon squash soft drink	58	17.0
Apple juice, mean of three studies	40	11.7
Carrot juice, freshly made	43	10.0
Cranberry juice drink	56	16.4
Grapefruit juice, unsweetened	48	10.7
Orange juice, mean of two studies	50	12.8
Pineapple juice, unsweetened	46	15.6
Tomato juice, canned	38	3.5
BREADS		
Baguette, white, plain	95	14.7
Barley kernel bread, mean of two studies	46	9.4
Hamburger bun	61	9.2
Gluten-free white bread, sliced (gluten-free wheat starch)	80	11.9
Wholegrain pumpernickel	46	5.2
Wholemeal rye bread, mean of four studies	58	8.4
White bread, mean of six studies	70	9.7
White bread with butter	59	28.5
Wholemeal bread, mean of thirteen studies	71	9.5
Soya and linseed loaf	36	3.2
Pita bread, white	57	9.5
BREAKFAST CEREALS		
All-Bran™ (Kellogg's)	38	8.7
Bran Flakes™ (Kellogg's)	74	13.2
Cornflakes, mean of five studies	81	20.8
Natural muesli, mean of two studies	49	9.6
Muesli, toasted	43	7.1
Nutrigrain™ (Kellogg's)	66	9.9
Porridge made from rolled oats, mean of eight studies	58	12.8
Puffed Wheat (Quaker Oats Co)	67	13.5
Raisin Bran™ (Kellogg's)	61	11.7
Rice Krispies™ (Kellogg's)	82	21.0
Shredded Wheat™ (Nabisco Brands Ltd)	83	16.6
Special K™ (Kellogg's)	54	11.3
Weetabix, mean of seven studies	70	13.0

CEREAL GRAINS

Amaranth eaten with milk and non-nutritive sweetener	97	21.0
Pearl barley, mean of five studies	25	10.6
Buckwheat, mean of three studies	54	16.1
Corn tortilla	52	12.4
Cornmeal (polenta), mean of two studies	69	9.0
Couscous, mean of two studies	65	22.7
Millet, boiled	71	25.2
Arborio, risotto rice, boiled	69	36.2
Boiled white rice, mean of 12 studies	64	23.3
Boiled long grain rice, mean of 10 studies	56	22.9
Glutinous rice, white, cooked in rice cooker	98	31.0
Jasmine rice, white, cooked in rice cooker	109	46.1
Basmati rice, white, boiled	58	21.8
Brown rice, mean of three studies	55	17.9
Rye, whole kernels, mean of three studies	34	12.9
Wheat, whole kernels, mean of four studies	41	14.0
Wheat tortilla (Mexican)	30	7.8
Bulgur wheat, mean of four studies	48	12.4

BISCUITS AND CRACKERS

Digestive biscuits, mean of three studies	59	9.7
Rich Tea biscuits	55	10.4
Shortbread	64	9.9
Rice cakes, mean of three studies	78	17.0
Ryvita, mean of four studies	64	10.5

DAIRY PRODUCTS AND ALTERNATIVES

Custard, home made from milk, wheat starch, and sugar	43	7.1
Ice cream, mean of five studies	61	7.9
Milk, full-fat, mean of five studies	27	3.1
Milk, skim	32	4.0
Milk, condensed, sweetened	61	17.0
Yoghurt	36	3.4
Low-fat, fruit yoghurt with aspartame	14	1.8
Soy milk, full-fat, 120 mg calcium	36	6.4
Soy yoghurt, peach and mango, 2% fat, sugar	50	13.0

FRUIT

Apples, raw, mean of six studies	38	5.5
Apricots, raw	57	5.2
Apricots, canned in light syrup	64	12.0
Apricots, dried (Australia)	30	8.0
Banana, mean of 10 studies	52	12.4
Cherries, raw	22	2.7
Dates, dried	103	41.6
Figs, dried	61	15.7
Grapefruit, raw	25	2.7
Grapes, mean of two studies	46	8.2
Kiwi fruit, mean of two studies	53	6.2
Lychee, canned in syrup and drained	79	16.1
Mango, mean of three studies	51	8.5
Oranges, mean of six studies	42	4.6
Papaya, mean of three studies	59	10.2
Peaches, mean of two studies	42	4.6
Peaches, canned, mean of two studies	38	4.2
Pears, raw, mean of four studies	38	4.2
Pineapple, mean of two studies	59	7.4
Plums, mean of two studies	39	4.8
Prunes	29	9.7
Raisins	64	28.5
Strawberries, fresh	40	1.3
Sultanas	56	25.2
Watermelon, raw	72	4.3

LEGUMES AND NUTS

Baked beans, canned, mean of two studies	48	7.4
Black beans	30	6.8
Blackeyed beans, boiled, mean of two studies	42	12.8
Butter beans, mean of three studies	31	6.1
Chickpeas, dried, boiled, mean of four studies	28	8.3
Haricot beans, mean of five studies	38	11.8
Kidney beans, mean of eight studies	28	6.9
Black beans, soaked overnight, cooked 45 min	20	4.9
Green lentils, mean of three studies	30	5.1
Red lentils, mean of four studies	26	4.8
Marrowfat peas, dried, boiled	47	7.4

Mung beans, germinated	25	4.3
Peas, dried, boiled	22	1.9
Pinto beans, dried, boiled	39	10.0
Soya beans, dried, boiled, mean of two studies	18	1.1
Soya beans, canned	14	0.8
Split peas, yellow, boiled 20 min	32	6.1

CONVENIENCE FOODS AND MIXED MEALS

Fish Fingers	38	7.3
Pizza, plain baked dough, served with Parmesan cheese and tomato sauce	80	21.6
Sirloin chop with mixed vegetables and mashed potato, home made	66	34.9
Spaghetti bolognaise, home made	52	25.0

PASTA AND NOODLES

Corn pasta, gluten-free	78	32.4
Gluten-free pasta, maize starch, boiled 8 min	54	22.5
Rice noodles, dried, boiled	61	23.5
Rice noodles, freshly made, boiled	40	15.4
Rice pasta, brown, boiled 16 min	92	34.8
Rice and maize pasta, gluten-free	76	36.9
Soba noodles, instant, reheated in hot water, served with soup	46	22.3
White spaghetti, boiled, mean of three cooking times	57	27.3
Wholemeal spaghetti, boiled, mean of two studies	37	15.5
Split pea and soya pasta shells, gluten-free	29	8.9
Udon noodles, plain, reheated 5 min	62	30.0
Vermicelli, white, boiled	35	15.5

SNACK FOODS AND CONFECTIONERY

Chocolate, milk, mean of four studies	43	12.0
Mars Bar®	68	27.1
Cashew nuts, salted	22	2.8
Peanuts, mean of three studies	14	0.8
Popcorn, mean of two studies	72	7.7
Potato crisps, mean of two studies	54	11.4
Snickers Bar®	68	23.1
Twix® Cookie Bar, caramel	44	17.0

SOUPS

Green pea soup, canned	66	27.3
Lentil soup, canned	44	9.0
Minestrone soup	39	7.1
Tomato soup	38	6.4

SUGARS

Honey, mean of 11 types	55	9.8

VEGETABLES

Peas, mean of three studies	48	3.4
Pumpkin	75	3.3
Sweet corn, mean of six studies	54	9.3
Beetroot	64	4.6
Carrots, raw	16	1.2
Cooked carrots, mean of four studies	47	2.7
Parsnips	97	12.1
Baked potato, mean of four studies	85	25.6
Boiled potatoes, mean of five studies	50	13.9
Mashed potato, mean of three studies	74	14.5
New potato, mean of three studies	57	12.0
Sweet potato, mean of five studies	61	17.0
Swede	72	7.5

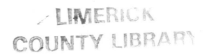

useful addresses

DIABETES ORGANISATIONS (INTERNATIONAL)

International Diabetes Federation

Executive Office
Avenue Emile De Mot 19
B-1000 Brussels
Belgium
Tel: +32-2-5385511
Fax: +32-2-5385114
info@idf.org
Website: www.idf.org
IDF publishes a Diabetes Atlas both online and in hard copy. The atlas covers epidemiology, economics, education, prevention, insulin and diabetes associations with a special emphasis on risk factors and primary prevention.

www.worlddiabetesfoundation.org

The World Diabetes Foundation is a charity registered in Denmark. It funds projects on diabetes awareness, education and capacity building at local, regional and global levels.

DIABETES ORGANISATIONS (UK)

Diabetes UK

10 Parkway
London NW1 7AA
Tel 020 7424 1000
Fax 020 7424 1001
Email info@diabetes.org.uk
Website: www.diabetes.org.uk
The leading charity working with people with diabetes.

Diabetes Research & Wellness Foundation

101-102 Northney Marina
Hayling Island
Hampshire PO11 0NH
Tel: 023 9263 7808
Fax: 023 9263 6137

Website: www.diabeteswellnessnet.org.uk
A registered charity, finances research into diabetes and supports people with diabetes through the Diabetes Wellness Network.

Juvenile Diabetes Research Foundation

25 Gosfield Street
London W1W 6EB
Tel: 020 7436 3112
Fax: 020 7436 3039
Website: www.jdrf.org.uk
Founded in 1986 by families living with diabetes, with the aim of finding a cure and improving the lives of their children.

DIABETES-RELATED WEBSITES

www.diabetes.org

The website of the American Diabetes Association. The mission of the Association is to prevent and cure diabetes.

www.diabetes.ca

The website of the Canadian Diabetes Association. Established over 50 years ago, the Canadian Diabetes Association promotes diabetes research, education, service and advocacy. A good interactive site.

www.diabetesindia.com

Diabetes India website, the aim of which is to provide people with diabetes and their treating physicians with the latest information thus giving them the power to control their diabetes.

www.diabetes-insight.info

The website of Diabetes Insight provides information for people and families with diabetes in the UK, to help them manage their diabetes and lead an active life. Email support group and excellent online forum.

www.mendosa.com

David Mendosa is a freelance medical writer and consultant specializing in diabetes. Free monthly email newsletter, Diabetes Update, and links to the latest diabetes research.

www.childrenwithdiabetes.com

American website for children, families and adults with diabetes. This website has a comprehensive list of national diabetes organisations in every country from Albania to Zambia.

www.healthtalk.com/den/

The Diabetes Education Network, a comprehensive source of information about diabetes

www.diabetesmonitor.com

A resource for patients to educate themselves about their role as active participants in the care of diabetes.

www.diabetesportal.com

A central one-stop resource for people with diabetes and their families.

http://members.tripod.com/diabetics_world/toc.htm.

Diabetics World is the website of Diabetics International Foundation. Its main objective is to disseminate information on diabetes and to stimulate interest in finding a cure.

FOOD INFORMATION AND FOOD SUPPLIERS

Abel & Cole

16 Waterside Way
Plough Lane
Wimbledon
London SW17 0HB
Tel: 08452 62 62 62
Fax: 020 8947 6662
Email: organics@abel-cole.co.uk
Website: www.abel-cole.co.uk.
Organic delivery service. Range of vegetable boxes, sustainably caught fish, organic meat and dairy products.

Aconbury Sprouts

Unit 4, Westwood Industrial Estate
Pontrilas
Hereford HR2 0EL
Tel/fax: 01981 241155
Email: info@aconbury.co.uk
Website: www.aconbury.co.uk
Beansprouts and wheatgrass. Online shopping available through the website.

Allied Bakeries

Vanwall Road
Maidenhead
SL6 4UF
Tel: 0870 1121 977
Email: info@burgen.co.uk
Suppliers of Burgen Soy Lin bread

Aquascot Group Limited

Fyrish Way
Alness
Highlands
Scotland IV17 0PJ
Tel: 01349 884481 Fax: 01349 883893
Email: service@aquascot.uk.com
Website: www.aquascot.com/organic.htm
Wholesale suppliers of organic salmon to Waitrose. Call for stockists.

Bacheldre Watermill

Churchstoke
Montgomery
Powys SY15 6TE
Tel: 01588 620489
Fax: 01588 620105
Email: info@bacheldremill.co.uk
Website: www.bacheldremill.co.uk
Suppliers of excellent quality organic stoneground flour

Big Oz Industries

PO Box 48
Twickenham
TW1 2UF
Tel: 020 8893 9366
Fax: 020 8893 8799
Email: enquiries@bigoz.co.uk
Website: www.bigoz.co.uk
Organic, gluten-free wholegrain cereals. Call for stockists.

Bioforce (UK) Ltd

2 Brewster Place
Irvine
Scotland KA11 5DD
Tel: 01294 277344
Fax: 01294 277922
Email: enquiries@bioforce.co.uk
Website: www.bioforce.co.uk
Suppliers of BioSnacky bean and seed mixtures for sprouting.

Cauldron Foods Ltd

Units 1-2
Portishead Business Park
Portishead
Bristol BS20 9BF
Tel: 01275 818448
Email: sandrat@cauldronfoods.co.uk
Website: www.cauldronfoods.co.uk
Vegetarian and organic convenience foods, including tofu. Call for stockists.

Clearspring Wholefoods Ltd

19A Acton Park Estate
London W3 7QE
Tel: 020 8749 1781
Website: www.clearspring.co.uk
Organic wholefoods from Japan, including shoyu, tamari and sea vegetables. Online shopping available through the website.

Coconut Oil UK

PO Box 11045
Dickens Heath
Solihull
West Midlands B90 1ZD
Tel: 0121 744 5753
Fax: 0121 744 5753
Email: info@coconut-oil-uk.com
Website: www.coconut-oil-uk.com
On-line shopping available on the website.

Daily Bread Co-operative

The Old Laundry
Bedford Road
Northampton
Tel: 01604 621531
Fax:- 01604 603725
Email: info@dailybread.co.uk
Website: www.dailybread.co.uk
Excellent value wholefood co-operative. Online ordering at www.ecofair.co.uk

Dove's Farm

Salisbury Road
Hungerford
Berkshire RG17 0RF
Tel: 01488 684 880
Fax: 01488 685 235
Email: portenquiry@dovesfarm.co.uk
Website: www.dovesfarm.co.uk
Organic and gluten-free flours, cereals and baked goods. Call for stockists.

Gilchesters Organic Farm

Hawkwell
Northumberland NE18 0QL
Tel: 01661 886119
Email info@gilchesters.com
Website: www.gilchesters.com
Organic wheat, spelt and rye flours, beef and lamb. Farm shop and mail order.

Graig Farm Organics

Dolau
Llandrindod Wells
Powys LD1 5TL
Telephone: 01597 851655
Fax: 01597 851991
Website: www.graigfarm.co.uk
One of the pioneers of organic meats and other organic foods in the UK. Mail order, availability through retail outlets and online ordering.

Hawkshead Trout Farm

The Boat House
Ridding Wood
Hawkshead
Ambleside
Cumbria LA22 0QF
Tel: 015394 36541
Fax: 015394 36541
Email: trout@hawkshead.demon.co.uk
Website: www.hawskhead.demon.co.uk
Suppliers of organic trout by mail order.

Marine Conservation Society (MCS)

Unit 3, Wolf Business Park
Alton Road
Ross-on-Wye
Herefordshire HR9 5NB
Tel: 01989 566017
Fax: 01989 567815
Website: www.mcsuk.org
Publishers of the Fish to Eat and Fish to Avoid lists at www.fishonline.org

Meridian Foods Ltd

Corwen
Clwyd
LL21 9RT
Tel: 01490 413151 Fax: 01490 412032
Email: info@meridianfoods.co.uk
Website: www.meridianfoods.co.uk
Suppliers of organic and special diet foods. Wholesale only. Call for stockists.

Orgran (UK) (Distributors)

Micross
Brent Terrace
London
NW2 1LT
www.orgran.com
Australian company supplying gluten-free and wheat-free pastas, crispbreads and snacks.

Riverford Organics Ltd

Wash Barn
Bukfastleigh
Devon TQ1 0LD
Tel: 01803 762720
Website: www.riverford.co.uk
Delivers organic boxes to the south of the UK. Affiliated box schemes from www.rivernene.co.uk (the Midlands) and www.riverswale.co.uk (the North).

Sanchi

PO Box 3577
London
NW2 1LQ
Email: info@sanchi.co.uk
Website: www.sanchi.co.uk
Shoyu and Tamari soy sauces, sea vegetables, miso, tofu and other Japanese products, available from health food shops.

Seagreens Limited

1 The Warren
Handcross
West Sussex
RH17 6DX
Tel: 01444 400403
Fax: 01444 400493
Email: post@seagreens.com
Website: www.seagreens.com
Seaweed granules for cooking and seaweed table condiment. Call for stockists.

Seasoned Pioneers

Unit 8 Stadium Court,
Stadium Road
Plantation Business Park
Bromborough
Wirral CH62 3RP
Tel: 0800 0682348
Email: feedback@seasonedpioneers.co.uk
Website: www.seasonedpioneers.co.uk
Suppliers of interesting spice mixes.

Simply Organic Food Company

Horsley Road
Kingsthorpe Hollow
Northampton NN2 6LJ
Tel: 0870 162 3010
Email: info@simplyorganic.net
Website: www.simplyorganic.net
Comprehensive organic mail-order service including fresh foods, groceries, personal and homecare products.

Suma Wholefoods

Lacy Way
Lowfields Business Park
Elland
West Yorkshire
HX5 9DB
Tel: 0845 458 2290
Fax: 0845 458 2295
Email: sales@suma.coop
Website: www.suma.co.uk
Independent wholesaler and distributor of
vegetarian, organic and natural foods. Call for
stockists.

Tilqhillie Fine Foods

Maryfield Farm
Tilquhillie
Banchory
Aberdeenshire AB31 6HY
Tel: 01330 822037 Fax: 01330 822037
Email: tillqpudds@tiscali.co.uk
Suppliers of guaranteed gluten-free oats,
puddings, muesli.

Whole Earth Foods Ltd

2 Valentine Place
London
SE1 8QH
Tel: 020 7633 5900
Fax: 020 7633 5901
Email: enquiries@wholeearthfoods.co.uk
Website: www.wholeearthfoods.co.uk
Organic drinks, cereals, spread, nut butters.
Call for stockists. Online shopping available on
the website.

Woodlands Park Dairy

Woodlands
Wimborne
Dorset BH21 8LX
Tel: 01202 822687 Fax: 01202 826051
Email: info@woodlands-park.co.uk
Website: www.woodlands-park.co.uk
Suppliers of goat's and sheep's milk yoghurt.

SUPPLEMENT COMPANIES

The Nutri Centre

7 Park Crescent
London W1N 3HE
Tel: 020 7436 5122
Fax: 020 7436 5171
Website: www.nutricentre.com
The Nutri Centre is situated on the lower
ground floor of the Hale Clinic. They are open to
the public and supply a very wide range of
supplements from many different companies as
well as an extensive selection of books on
nutrition and health. On-line shopping available
on their website.

BioCare Ltd

Lakeside
180 Lifford Lane
Kings Norton
Birmingham B30 3NU
Tel: 0121 433 3727
Fax: 0121 433 3879
Email: biocare@biocare.co.uk
Website: www.biocare.co.uk
Innovative company originally founded by
practitioners for practitioners. Product range
available from The Nutri Centre and selected
healthcare stores.

Higher Nature

The Nutrition Centre
Burwash Common
East Sussex
TN19 7LX
Tel: 01435 884 668
Fax: 01435 883720
Email: info@higher-nature.co.uk
Website: www.highernature.co.uk
Online shopping available on the website.
Product range also available from The Nutri
Centre. Suppliers of Omega organic coconut
oil.

index

index

notes

notes

notes

notes

notes

notes